# NON-INVASIVE VENTILATION MADE SIMPLE

GW00566696

# Non-Invasive Ventilation Made Simple

Dr William J.M. Kinnear
*University Hospital, Nottingham*

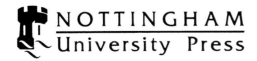

NOTTINGHAM
University Press

Nottingham University Press
Manor Farm, Main Street, Thrumpton
Nottingham, NG11 0AX, United Kingdom

NOTTINGHAM

First published 2007
Reprinted 2009
© WJM Kinnear

**British Library Cataloguing in Publication Data**

*Disclaimer*

# Contents

For Sue, Anne and Katie

# Abbreviations

| | |
|---|---|
| AMU | acute medicine unit |
| ARDS | adult respiratory distress syndrome |
| ASB | assisted spontaneous breathing |
| AVAPS | average volume-assured pressure support |
| BIPAP | bi-level positive airway pressure |
| BP | blood pressure |
| CF | cystic fibrosis |
| $cmH_2O$ | centimetres of water |
| $CO_2$ | carbon dioxide |
| COPD | chronic obstructive pulmonary disease |
| CPAP | continuous positive airway pressure |
| CSF | cerebrospinal fluid |
| CXR | chest X-ray |
| ED | emergency department |
| EPAP | expiratory positive airway pressure |
| ET | endo-tracheal |
| FEV1 | forced expired volume in one second |
| GCS | Glasgow coma scale |
| HDU | high dependency unit |
| HME | heat and moisture exchanger |
| ICU | intensive care unit |
| I:E | inspiratory:expiratory |
| IPAP | inspiratory positive airway pressure |
| IPPV | intermittent positive pressure ventilation |
| kPa | kilopascal |
| L | litre |
| LVF | left ventricular failure |
| MEP | maximum expiratory mouth pressure |
| MIP | maximum inspiratory mouth pressure |
| Ml | millilitre |
| mmHg | millimeters of mercury |
| MND | motor neurone disease |
| NIPPV | non-invasive intermittent positive pressure ventilation |
| NIV | non-invasive ventilation |
| $O_2$ | oxygen |
| $PaCO_2$ | arterial partial pressure of carbon dioxide |
| $PaO_2$ | arterial partial pressure of oxygen |
| $PAO_2$ | alveolar partial pressure of oxygen |
| PCF | peak cough flow |
| PEEPi | intrinsic positive end-expiratory pressure |
| PEFR | peak expiratory flow rate |
| RCT | randomised controlled trial |
| RR | respiratory rate |
| SNIP | sniff nasal inspiratory pressure |
| $SaO_2$ | arterial oxygen saturation |
| SARS | severe acute respiratory syndrome |
| $SpO_2$ | peripheral oxygen saturation |
| TB | tuberculosis |
| Ti | inspiratory time |
| TTI | tension time index |
| Ttot | total breath time |
| VC | vital capacity |
| Vt | tidal volume |

# Keywords

**Alveolar hypoventilation:** Reduced ventilation of the gas-exchanging part of the lungs, with inadequate elimination of $CO_2$.

**Aspiration**: Inhalation of gastric contents into the lungs.

**Assist:** When the ventilator helps the patient's spontaneous breathing pattern.

**Autotriggering:** Triggering of the ventilator when it is not connected to the patient, caused by high flow of air down the circuit.

**Bi-level positive airway pressure:** The commonest mode of pressure-support non-invasive ventilation, combining inspiratory and expiratory positive airway pressure.

**Central hypoventilation:** Type 2 respiratory failure caused by poor respiratory drive.

**Control:** When the ventilator delivers breaths to the patient independently of their breathing pattern.

**Expiratory positive airway pressure:** Positive pressure applied to the airway during expiration.

**Fractional inspired oxygen:** The concentration of oxygen a patient breaths in.

**Hypercapnia:** Elevated arterial carbon dioxide level.

**Hypoxia:** Low arterial oxygen level - strictly speaking, the correct term is hypoxaemia.

**Inspiratory positive airway pressure:** Positive pressure applied to the airway during inspiration.

**Inspiratory:expiratory ratio**: The ratio of the time spent in inspiration to that in expiration.

**Interface:** The device used to connect the ventilator to the patient.

**Intrinsic positive end-expiratory pressure:** Pressure inside the thorax when the lungs are unable to empty completely.

**Intubation:** Insertion of an endotracheal tube to provide "invasive" ventilation.

**Non-invasive intermittent positive pressure ventilation:** The commonest pressure-control mode of non-invasive ventilation.

**Non-invasive ventilation:** Artificial ventilation that doesn't use an endotracheal tube or tracheostomy.

**Pressure control ventilation:** NIV where you set the pressure and the timing of breaths.

**Pressure support ventilation**: NIV where the only thing you set is the pressure – the patient determines the timing.

**Pressure-targeted ventilation:** NIV where you set the target pressure for each breath.

**Obesity-hypoventilation syndrome:** Chronic type 2 respiratory failure in very obese patients

**Rebreathing**: The patient inhales air they have just breathed out.

**Respiratory acidosis**: Elevation of the $PaCO_2$ with a low pH level.

**Rise time**: The time taken at the start of inspiration to reach the target pressure.

**Scoliosis:** Curvature of the spine.

**Span:** The difference between IPAP and EPAP.

**Tidal volume:** The volume of air entering the lungs with each breath.

**Type 1 respiratory failure:** Failure of oxygenation, with a normal or low $PaCO_2$.

**Type 2 respiratory failure:** Failure of ventilation, with an elevated $PaCO_2$.

**Vital capacity:** The maximum amount of air a patient can take in – or blow out - with a single breath.

**Volume-targeted ventilation:** NIV where you set the target tidal volume for each breath, rather than the pressure.

**Weaning:** The gradual reduction of ventilatory support until either the patient is breathing independently or further reduction cannot be achieved.

**Work of breathing:** The amount of energy used in moving air in and out of the lungs.

# 1

# Background

**Learning points:**

By the end of this chapter you should be able to:

- Describe the difference between non-invasive ventilation (NIV) and invasive ventilation.

- List a few different places where NIV might be used.

- Explain why you think you need to know about NIV.

- *Compare patients who might need NIV acutely with those who use it long term at home.*

**Keywords**:

Non-invasive ventilation, Bi-level positive airway pressure (BIPAP), Non-invasive intermittent positive pressure ventilation (NIPPV).

## What is "Non-invasive" ventilation?

*Key points*

NIV uses positive pressure to inflate the lungs, but with a mask rather than an endotracheal tube.

When we talk about a patient being "ventilated", we usually mean artificial ventilation provided by a life-support machine or ventilator. Sometimes this is called mechanical ventilation. "Invasive" in this context means the ventilator is connected to an endotracheal tube or tracheostomy. There are a few other ways of providing artificial ventilation which are non-invasive - iron lungs, cuirasses, pneumobelts, rocking beds, etc. Their use is largely confined to specialist centres and we won't discuss them further.

1

In this book, the term "NIV" includes the two commonest modes of NIV, both of which use positive pressure to inflate the lungs:

- BIPAP (bi-level positive airway pressure) is a form of pressure support, whereby the patient breathes spontaneously and the ventilator provides some supporting pressure with each breath.

- NIPPV (non-invasive positive pressure ventilation) is called pressure control, because the ventilator rather than the patient controls both the rate and the pattern of breathing.

Don't worry too much about the difference between these modes at this stage – we'll spend time on this topic at various points in the book.

Continuous positive airway pressure (CPAP) can be used to improve oxygenation, or to keep the upper airway patent. Although the same sorts of mask are used, it is not really a form of ventilation.

## Why do I need to know about NIV?

- On the intensive care unit (ICU), NIV is used as a primary treatment for respiratory failure and also to help wean from invasive ventilation. Even if you are fully conversant with the sorts of ventilators used for invasive ventilation, there are some important aspects of NIV which you need to understand.

- For every 100,000 people in the population, there will be between 5 and 10 patients who use NIV at home, often just at night. They may develop acute respiratory failure - for example when they get a chest infection - and need admission to hospital. You may also want to know more if you are likely to come across these patients in clinics or in the community.

## What do I need to know about NIV?

A ventilator is usually thought of as a piece of equipment used in the operating theatre or on an ICU. It will have lots of control knobs and dials. Working these is best left to an anaesthetist or intensivist. Non-invasive ventilators are much simpler and easier to use.

There are several themes running through this book: the equipment you need for NIV, the patients you will be treating, simple physiology and practical tips. Everything you need to know should be included at some point. At the start of each chapter there is an indication of what is covered (with some keywords which you will find defined at the beginning of the book); more advanced learning points are in italics and refer to the later sections of each chapter. A thick line across the text tells you when you are about to enter the more complicated sections:

===============================================================

You might decide to skip on to the next chapter when you get to this line the first time you read through the book, particularly if you are new to NIV and find the amount of information a bit daunting.

I have worked on the assumption that you are likely to read through this book once, then come back to it for reference. The technical, clinical and theoretical topics are mixed together, in the hope of an easier and more enjoyable to read. It should still be simple to refer back to a particular topic.

In this chapter you have already come across Learning Points, Keywords and a Key Point. The other highlighted sections are Terminology, Practical Tips, How To Do It and Physiology.

## Summary

- NIV is artificial ventilation using a mask rather than an endotracheal tube.
- NIV is used widely in many different acute situations - you need to know something about it if you work in an acute hospital.
- NIV is much simpler to manage than invasive ventilation on ICU.
- Quite a few patients use NIV at home, often just at night.

# 2
# Building Blocks

**Learning points**:

By the end of this chapter you should be able to:

* Draw a block diagram showing the three main components of NIV.
* *Explain why mask leaks are such a problem.*

A patient with an exacerbation of their chronic obstructive pulmonary disease (COPD) comes into hospital with acute hypercapnic respiratory failure. They aren't improving despite optimal drug therapy and controlled oxygen. You decide they need NIV: you will need a pump (the ventilator), an interface (the mask) and tubing to connect the two together (the circuit):

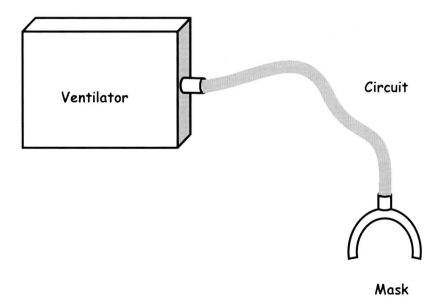

**Figure 2.1** The three components of NIV: a ventilator, connected by circuit tubing to a mask.

## The pump

The pump is a simple piece of equipment which contains a fan (or sometimes bellows) to deliver air to the patient. There are different ways of setting up the pump - we will discuss these in detail later on. All we need for the moment is something that will deliver air under positive pressure. We won't spend time looking at individual makes of ventilator, as new designs come along every year.

### Practical Tip

Use a ventilator specifically designed for NIV.

Standard ICU ventilators tend not to be very good at NIV, because they were designed for use with an endotracheal tube and can't cope with the leaks that are inevitable with a mask.

## The circuit

The circuit is also simple - a length of tubing usually about a metre or so long. It needs to be long enough to allow the patient to move around in bed; if it is too long then the ventilator may struggle with the resistance to flow. The tube should be wide bore to allow the air to flow freely into the patient – about 22mm in diameter, similar to the "elephant" tubing you may have used to deliver high-flow oxygen on the wards. Tubing with a smooth internal surface offers the least resistance to flow, but corrugated tubing is fine for most NIV purposes. We will need some holes and valves depending upon the way we use NIV, but we'll discuss these later. In essence, the circuit is a wide bore tube which takes the air from the ventilator to the patient.

## The mask

The mask is the crucial thing about NIV. Getting a mask to fit well is the most skilful bit. It needs to be comfortable for the patient. There must be a good enough seal so that most of the air from the ventilator goes into the patient rather than leaking around the edges of the mask.

### Key points

NIV is all about getting the mask to fit well.

## Leaks

The main problem with NIV is managing leaks. You will spend a lot of time adjusting masks to try and minimise leaks. Leaks mean that ventilators have to work harder to get the mask up to the required pressure, they don't know how much of the air they delivered in a breath has gone into the patient and how much has leaked into the room (which is why we tend not to use ventilators on which we only set the volume of each breath, or tidal volume) and it is more difficult for them to work out when the patient wants to breathe. During sleep, leaks around the mask and through the mouth are the main reason that nocturnal hypoventilation persists despite NIV. Air leaking around the mask blows into the patient's eyes, makes a noise and is generally uncomfortable.

### *Terminology*

**PaO$_2$ and PaCO$_2$**

NIV is used to treat respiratory failure. To decide whether or not a patient is in respiratory failure, we need to know about their oxygen and carbon dioxide levels. This usually requires an arterial blood gas sample, on which we measure the amount of oxygen (PaO$_2$) and carbon dioxide (PaCO$_2$) - the "P" stands for partial pressure. PaCO$_2$ should be less than 6kPa (or 45mmHg). PaO$_2$ declines with age. The normal range for PaO$_2$ is 10-13kPa (76-100mmHg), although values at the lower end of this range are only normal in the elderly.

## Pulse oximetry

One basic piece of equipment you are likely to use with NIV is a pulse oximeter - a simple finger probe that tells you what the patient's peripheral oxygen saturation is. This is called SpO$_2$ (as opposed to SaO$_2$, which is the saturation of an arterial sample measured using a blood gas machine). Although oximeters don't give us any direct information about carbon dioxide, their wide availability and ease of use means that we'll be using them to assess and monitor patients during NIV.

### *Practical Tip*

When you take an arterial blood gas sample, you should see it pulsate into the sample syringe - if you don't and are worried that it might be venous, just compare the SaO$_2$ of the sample with SpO$_2$. If they are very different, you need to repeat the blood gas. It is all too common to see "?venous – repeat" written on very abnormal blood gas results, when simple comparison with the SpO$_2$ will confirm that the patient is very unwell and needs urgent intervention.

## Summary

- NIV uses an air pump (ventilator), connected by a tube (circuit) to a mask (interface).
- Fitting the mask is the skilful bit.

# 3

# Basic Principles

---

## Learning points:

By the end of this chapter you should be able to:

- Draw a graph showing how airway pressure increases and decreases during NIV.

- *Draw a graph of inspiratory flow during NIV, and explain why flow tails off towards the end of inspiration.*

## Keywords:

Inspiratory positive airway pressure (IPAP), Pressure-targeted ventilation, Tidal volume (Vt).

---

## Pressure

Think of the lung as a balloon. To expand the balloon in the way that NIV expands the chest, we need to blow air in. Imagine blowing into the balloon, and then taking your mouth away to let the air flow out again as the balloon collapses - for the sake of simplicity, this is a very small balloon that you can blow up in one breath. If we measured the pressure in the balloon as you blew into it, there would be a positive pressure, say $15cmH_2O$ which is a common starting pressure for NIV. When you took your mouth away, the balloon would deflate and the pressure would return to zero (atmospheric). This is the principle of NIV, except that instead of you blowing up a balloon there is a ventilator blowing air into a patient. The pressure trace would look like figure 3.1.

### Terminology

#### IPAP

The pressure we use to inflate the lungs is applied during inspiration and so is called Inspiratory Positive Airway Pressure, or IPAP.

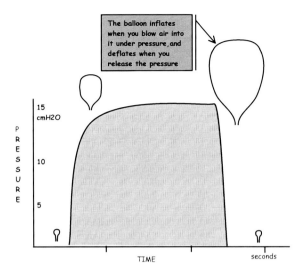

**Figure 3.1** Pressure-time trace for a single inspiration of NIV.

## Flow

The chest becomes more and more difficult to inflate as you blow more air into it. You can feel this yourself: as you start a breath it is quite easy to get air in, but if you breathe right up to your full lung capacity then it is much more difficult towards the end. We could record this as flow. At the beginning of the breath the flow of air into the lungs is high, but it tails off:

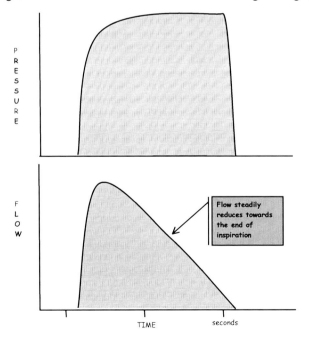

**Figure 3.2** Flow-time trace of a single inspiration on NIV.

On a ventilator flow trace, you will probably also see expiratory flow:

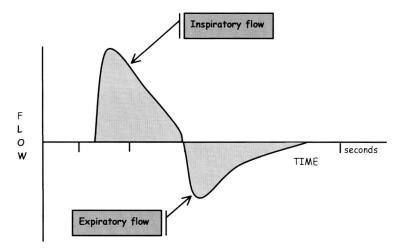

Figure 3.3 Inspiratory and expiratory flow of a single breath on NIV.

## Volume

Air flowing into the lungs leads to an increase in volume. Since flow is highest at the start of inspiration, the increase in volume is steepest at this point. During expiration, the volume of the lungs decreases again:

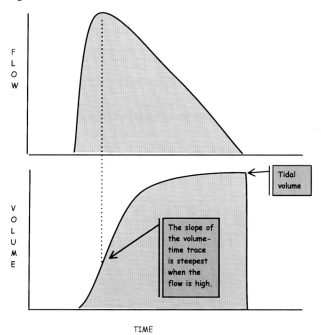

Figure 3.4 Flow and volume trace for a single inspiration on NIV.

The volume entering the lungs with each breath is called Tidal Volume (Vt).  If we look at the pressure-volume curve of the lungs, the more pressure we use to inflate the lungs, the greater the volume they will expand to:

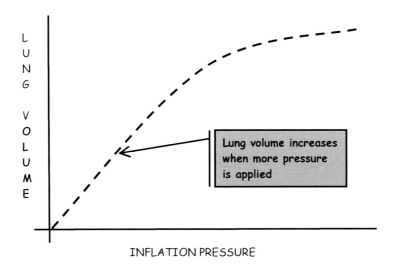

LUNG VOLUME

Lung volume increases when more pressure is applied

INFLATION PRESSURE

**Figure 3.5** Pressure-volume curve of the lungs.

The same applies to NIV - the higher the IPAP you use, the greater Vt you will get.  We'll return to this pressure-volume curve at several points in the book.

*Terminology*

**Pressure-targeted ventilation**

In our balloon example, we aimed for a pressure of 15cmH$_2$O.  This is the target pressure which we set on the ventilator.  Both BIPAP and NIPPV are pressure-targeted modes of ventilation.

## Summary

- NIV uses positive pressure to push air into the chest.
- This is like blowing up a balloon.
- The flow into the chest is high at the start of a breath in, then tails off.
- Higher pressures generate larger volumes.

# 4

# Masks

---

**Learning points**:

By the end of this chapter you should be able to:

- Decide whether to use a nasal or full-face mask for NIV.

- Choose a mask of an appropriate size.

- Demonstrate how you would fit the mask to the patient.

- *Explain when you would use other interfaces such as mouthpieces and helmets.*

**Keywords**:

Interface

---

The most crucial aspect of NIV is the "interface" between the ventilator and the patient. This is usually a mask, but there are a few other options to consider such as nasal pillows, mouthpieces and helmets.

## Oronasal masks

If you get breathless, you tend to breathe through your mouth. For this reason, in most acute situations a mask which covers the nose and mouth is the best option to try first. The mask has a cushioned edge to form a seal with the face. You may need to try several sizes on the patient before you get the best fit. When you strap the mask in place, tighten the straps as tight as is necessary to prevent leaks – if this is intolerably tight for the patient, try a different size of mask. If this doesn't work, try a nasal mask.

> **Key points**
>
> NIV masks are very different from oxygen masks – they fit much more tightly to the face in order to achieve a seal.

## Nasal masks

Face masks tend to move around a bit. This isn't surprising considering how mobile our jaws are. A nasal mask is much more stable on the bones of the face. For patients starting NIV in a non-acute setting, a nasal mask is often the best choice to try first.

**Practical Tip**

In acute respiratory failure in adults, start with a mask which covers the mouth and nose. In less acute situations, or in children, start with a nasal mask.

Smaller masks tend to work better than larger ones. Keep the patient's dentures in (unless their consciousness is impaired): the mask will tend to stay in place better. You might think when a ventilator is attached to a mask over the nose, the air would come straight out the mouth. In practice, patients quickly learn to use their soft palate to block off the connection between their nose and mouth, and the ventilator works fine. Some patients get the hang of this quite quickly, a few never manage it.

**How to do it**

**Reduce mask leaks:**

- Pull the mask slightly away from the face, centre it and "re-bed" it on the patient.
- Press gently on the mask and see if this reduces the leak; if so, tighten the straps slightly. Over-tightening the straps makes the mask uncomfortable without reducing leakage much.
- Change to a smaller mask.
- Try a different style of mask.
- Try an individually moulded mask, if you have them available.
- Reduce the airway pressure. The patient will get less ventilation, but if it means they will tolerate NIV better then you may accept this.
- If air is leaking from the mouth with a nasal mask, use a chin strap or change to a mask which covers the mouth.

## Infection control

In acute respiratory failure, masks should be used on one patient and then discarded. For longer term use at home, masks will last about six months if cared for well. They should be dismantled and washed in warm soapy water daily.

**Practical Tip**

NIV masks and circuits that look clean are unlikely to be a source of infection.

## Nasal pillows

Nasal pillows, or cushions, consist of soft pads that fit just inside the patient's nostrils. They are attached to a rigid plastic tube which comes up over the forehead to the headgear. They are less claustrophobic than a mask, and it is often easier to set them up without putting any pressure on the nasal bridge. The only down side is that they can be prone to displacement if the patient is moving around a lot. Many patients like to use nasal pillows for daytime NIV, because they can see better than with a mask. Even better in this regard are the nasal cannulae designed for NIV, with large soft ends which fit tightly inside the nostrils.

### Practical Tip

If the bridge of the patient's nose starts to get red from mask pressure, change to a different mask or use an alternative device such as nasal pillows.

## Mouthpieces

You can also use a mouthpiece for patients who need to use NIV during the daytime, for example patients with neuromuscular diseases. This could be a simple mouthpiece such as that sometimes used with a nebulizer, if the patient needs only a few breaths of NIV now and then. A flanged mouthpiece may be better if NIV is needed for slightly longer periods. It is possible to use a mouthpiece for overnight NIV – some patients with neuromuscular disorders affecting their arms or hands may find it easier to set themselves up on NIV if they use a mouthpiece rather than a mask.

## Helmets

Helmets which fit right over the patient's head can sometimes be useful in acute respiratory failure. Breathless patients may tolerate them better than a mask. You need higher pressures than for masks, on account of the large volume of the helmet.

## What should you keep in stock?

If you are starting an acute NIV service, see if there are any anaesthetic face masks already in use on your unit which are being used for CPAP. If they are any good, stick with these but make sure you have at least three different sizes. If you are already using nasal masks to treat obstructive sleep apnoea, it probably makes sense to stick with the same style - make sure you have at least five different sizes, including some very small ones. My next choice would be a few sets of nasal pillows, to get you out of trouble if pressure over the bridge of the nose starts to damage the skin. Most units have a variety of different makes of face and nasal masks in stock. Some patients find different styles more comfortable. If you can't get a good fit with the first two or three you try then you are likely to end up trying every mask you have.

## Summary

- Use a full face mask first in acute respiratory failure.

- Use a nasal mask first in chronic respiratory failure.

- You'll need to keep quite a wide selection in stock.

- Nasal pillows, nasal cannulae, mouthpieces and helmets are alternatives to masks which are sometimes useful.

# 5

# Respiratory Failure

**Learning points**:

By the end of this chapter you should be able to

- Distinguish between type 1 and type 2 respiratory failure.
- List three reasons why a patient might develop type 2 respiratory failure.
- *Work out from some blood gas results whether type 2 respiratory failure is acute or chronic.*
- *Explain why NIV tends to work best in type 2 respiratory failure.*
- *Define FiO$_2$.*

## Keywords:

Alveolar hypoventilation, FiO$_2$, Respiratory acidosis, Type 1 and type 2 respiratory failure, Work of breathing.

## Type 1 and type 2 respiratory failure

Before we start using NIV, let's pause to think in a little more detail about respiratory failure. Most of the evidence for the effectiveness of NIV is in patients with type 2 respiratory failure. What does type 2 mean?

In type 2 respiratory failure there isn't enough air getting to the gas-exchanging part of the lungs. Carbon dioxide isn't removed effectively, so the PaCO$_2$ rises.

In type 2 respiratory failure the PaO$_2$ will be low, unless the patient is breathing supplementary oxygen, but the main issue is failure of ventilation rather than oxygenation.

---

**Terminology**

**Inspired oxygen concentration**

You will come across the term $FiO_2$. This means the **F**raction of the **i**nspired gas that is oxygen. As you know, about 21% of air is oxygen, so the $FiO_2$ would be 0.21. A patient breathing 60% oxygen has an $FiO_2$ of 0.60. Sometimes $FiO_2$ is written as a percent (eg $FiO_2 = 60\%$), which is a bit confusing.

## Causes of type 2 (hypercapnic) respiratory failure

Type 2 respiratory failure develops in three main situations:

- The **work** asked of the respiratory muscles is too great for them to sustain. An example of this would be a patient with a deformed ribcage which means it is stiff which makes it difficult for the respiratory muscles to expand.
- The respiratory **muscles** are weak, and unable to ventilate the lungs. This is what happens in muscular dystrophy.
- Central respiratory **drive** is impaired, and the respiratory muscles aren't told to ventilate the lungs. Poor central drive is seen with some diseases of the central nervous system and in the obesity-hypoventilation syndrome.

I like the analogy which is sometimes used of a person who has to carry a box across a room. They might fail because the box is too heavy, because they are weak, or because their motivation (or drive) to do the task is not high. It is quite common for there to be some contribution from more than one of these three aspects: in COPD, lots of ventilation is wasted in parts of the lung that don't exchange gas well (dead-space), so the work of breathing is high; the inspiratory muscles don't work very effectively because the chest is at such a high lung volume; many COPD patients have poor respiratory drive (they are sometimes called "blue bloaters" because they are cyanosed, overweight and oedematous).

## Alveolar ventilation and dead space

Total ventilation is the amount of air going in and out of the lungs. You calculate this by multiplying the breathing rate by the size of each breath (Vt). The result is expressed in litres per minute. Some of this ventilation is "wasted" on dead space. Dead space has two components:

- Parts of the lung which do not have alveoli, such as the trachea and bronchi.
- Parts which do have alveoli but they do not exchange gas with the blood particularly well.

The bit without alveoli is called "anatomical" dead space, but we are much more interested in the total amount of wasted ventilation – called "physiological" dead space.

The amount of ventilation getting to the gas-exchanging part of the lungs is called "alveolar ventilation" and is calculated as follows:

Breathing Rate x (Tidal Volume – Physiological Dead Space)

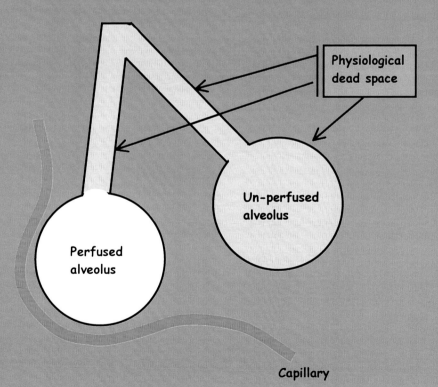

**Figure 5.1** Physiological dead space, which includes underperfused alveoli.

## Acute or chronic?

Elevation of $PaCO_2$ is called hypercapnia, and the next thing we need to decide is whether the patient has acute or chronic hypercapnia. This is quite important in COPD, because NIV works best when the $PaCO_2$ has gone up during an acute illness or exacerbation. $CO_2$ in the blood combines with water ($H_2O$) to create carbonic acid ($H_2CO_3$), which dissociates into bicarbonate ($HCO_3^-$) and hydrogen ($H^+$):

$$CO_2 + H_2O = H_2CO_3 = H^+ + HCO_3^-$$

$H^+$ is an acid. This is a "respiratory" acidosis because the cause is $CO_2$, as opposed to a "metabolic" acidosis where the acid comes from somewhere else (ketones or lactate for example). Acidosis is a low pH level – less than 7.35 (or a high hydrogen ion concentration, if you use this instead of pH).

The pH level is related to the ratio of $HCO_3^-$ to $CO_2$. In a respiratory acidosis – where there is too much $CO_2$ - the kidneys will try to get the pH back to normal by increasing the concentration of bicarbonate. This compensatory mechanism is of more relevance in some diseases than others. For example, you will probably want to consider NIV in a patient with muscular dystrophy who is hypercapnic, irrespective of the pH level. In COPD, NIV works mainly in acute hypercapnic respiratory failure, when the pH level will be low.

> ### *Key point*
>
> In respiratory acidosis, the $PaCO_2$ is greater than 6kPa (45mmHg) and the pH level is less than 7.35. If the bicarbonate is greater than 30mmol/litre then the $PaCO_2$ has been high for some time – probably several days or more.

## Type 1 respiratory failure

In type 1 respiratory failure, there is plenty of air getting into the lungs, but they are not very effective in getting oxygen from the air across into the bloodstream. The $PaO_2$ is therefore low. It is much easier to wash carbon dioxide out than it is to get oxygen in, so in Type 1 respiratory failure the $PaCO_2$ is normal – it may even be low if the patient hyperventilates in an attempt to get more oxygen in.

> ### *Key point*
>
> Type 2 respiratory failure is a failure of <u>ventilation</u>, hence non-invasive <u>ventilation</u> tends to work well. Type 1 respiratory failure is failure of oxygenation rather than ventilation, and NIV is less effective.

The physiology of hypoxia is quite complex, but the most important process is the mis-matching of ventilation and perfusion. For the moment it is sufficient to say that type 1 respiratory failure is failure of oxygenation and indicates lung disease. The more severe the hypoxia, the less likely the patient is to benefit from NIV (which is also true in type 2 respiratory failure).

*How to do it*

**Diagnose respiratory failure from arterial blood gases**

- Check what $FiO_2$ the patient was breathing when the sample was taken.
- Is the $PaO_2$ low? This depends on age and $FiO_2$.
- Is the $PaCO_2$ > 6kPa (45mmHg) ? If it is, then this is type 2 respiratory failure.
- Is the pH level less than 7.35? If the $PaCO_2$ is high and the pH level is low, this is a respiratory acidosis.
- Is the $HCO_3^-$ > 30mmol/L? If it is, this is a chronic respiratory acidosis.
- Ignore all the other bits of data that are invariably printed out on the report – they don't add anything to the diagnosis of respiratory failure.

## Summary

- Type 2 respiratory failure is an elevated $PaCO_2$

- A low pH level indicates that the high $PaCO_2$ is an acute problem that the kidneys have not yet had time to compensate for

- NIV works best in type 2 respiratory failure

- In both types of respiratory failure, the more hypoxic the patient is, the less likely they are to benefit from NIV

# 6
# Modes of Ventilation

---

## Learning points:

By the end of this chapter you should be able to:

* Define pressure support ventilation.

* Draw a graph showing how inspiratory and expiratory pressure combine to provide BIPAP.

* *Differentiate between BIPAP and NIPPV.*

* *Explain how pressure control differs from pressure support.*

* *Outline the difference between flow-cycling and time-cycling.*

## Keywords:

Expiratory positive airway pressure (EPAP), Pressure-control ventilation, Pressure-support ventilation.

---

There are dozens of different modes of ventilation. As we have mentioned already, you only really need to know in detail about two – pressure support (BIPAP) and pressure control (NIPPV).

## Pressure support ventilation

In pressure support ventilation, the only thing we set is the level of pressure that the ventilator will deliver with each breath. The timing is determined by the patient, who triggers the beginning and end of each breath. Pressure support is so-called because the patient is breathing spontaneously with their own breathing rhythm, but with each breath they are being helped (supported) to breathe in by the IPAP from the ventilator. In an acute situation, the patient's breathing rate and pattern are liable to change as they get better. The beauty of pressure support is that the ventilator will follow any changes, without you having to continually adjust the rate and inspiratory:expiratory (I:E) ratio. There is usually a back-up setting if the patient's breathing becomes too slow, and you do have to set the rate and I:E ratio for that - we'll come back to this later.

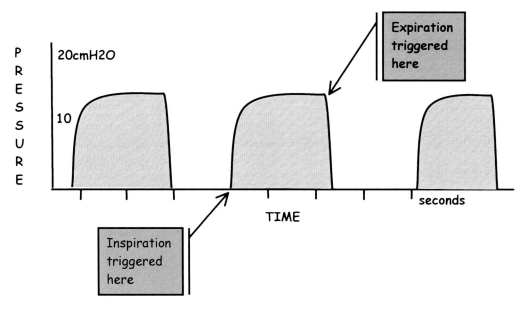

**Figure 6.1** Pressure-time trace of three breaths during pressure support ventilation. The patient triggers each breath, so the interval between breaths is variable. The target pressure of 12cmH$_2$O is the same for each breath, but they are of different lengths, since the patient also triggers the switch across into expiration.

## Bi-level pressure support (BIPAP)

CPAP is used in ICU or HDU to keep the lungs fully expanded, for example in patients with pneumonia, and to provide a bit of extra pressure to help with the transfer of oxygen across into the blood stream. CPAP involves application of the same pressure throughout the breathing cycle. It is also used in the treatment of obstructive sleep apnoea, to keep the upper airway open during sleep. The pressure-time trace during CPAP looks like this:

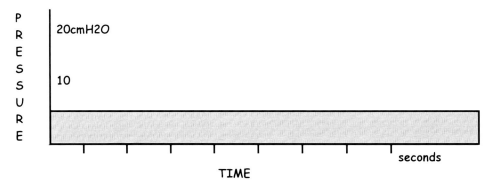

**Figure 6.2** Pressure-time trace of CPAP at 5cmH$_2$O.

If we combine pressure support and CPAP, we get a high pressure during inspiration (IPAP) with a lower background pressure during expiration. The background pressure is no longer called CPAP (because it is not "continuous") but becomes EPAP - expiratory positive airway pressure:

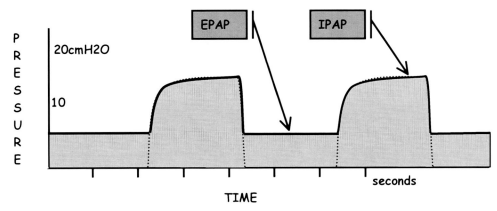

**Figure 6.3** Pressure-time trace of two breaths during bilevel pressure support ventilation (BIPAP), with an IPAP of 15cmH$_2$O and an EPAP of 5cmH$_2$O.

Adding EPAP has some physiological advantages, as we'll discuss later on. One useful effect of EPAP is that it allows us to use a very simple circuit – we'll see why in the next chapter. "Bi-level pressure support" doesn't exactly trip off the tongue, so let's use the commonly-used term "BIPAP" (short for bi-level positive airway pressure - in ICU this mode is sometimes called "CPAP/ASB" with ASB standing for assisted spontaneous breathing.)

> ***Terminology***
>
> BIPAP is bi-level pressure support. It is the most widely used mode for treating acute respiratory failure

## Bi-level pressure control

With some ventilators, we could allow the patient to decide when they start each breath, but insist that the breath cannot be shorter than a specified time – say two seconds. We are now moving towards controlling breathing rather than supporting it. The advantage of setting a minimum time for inspiration is in preventing the patient from taking very rapid shallow breaths, which is inefficient in terms of gas exchange. You would also arrive at the same sort of mode by starting NIPPV (see next section) and then deciding to add some CPAP. Confusingly, in ICU this sort of pressure-control is sometimes called BIPAP. Just to clarify things, in this book BIPAP refers to bi-level pressure support, with the patient determining the timing of breaths.

## Pressure control (NIPPV)

The most common pressure-control mode is non-invasive intermittent positive pressure ventilation (NIPPV). It is the mode used by many patients on long-term ventilation at home, and is also sometimes needed for acute respiratory failure, for example if BIPAP fails or in patients with ventilatory pump problems (drive, muscle or chest wall problems). At the risk of labouring the point, and perhaps of over-simplification, you could think of BIPAP as <u>supporting</u> ventilation and NIPPV as <u>delivering</u> ventilation.

The features of NIPPV are as follows:

- Like BIPAP, NIPPV is a pressure-targeted mode - the ventilator is set to deliver the same pressure with each breath.

- An exhalation valve in the circuit opens at the end of inspiration, so that the pressure during expiration falls to zero.

- The duration of inspiration is set (or "controlled").

- The respiratory rate is set. This is not just a back-up rate: the patient will be ventilated at this rate most of the time.

- The patient can trigger a breath, but they usually don't. If they do, it will be the same duration as an untriggered breath.

In the example below, the third breath is triggered slightly early by the patient, but you should be able to see that it looks like all the other breaths:

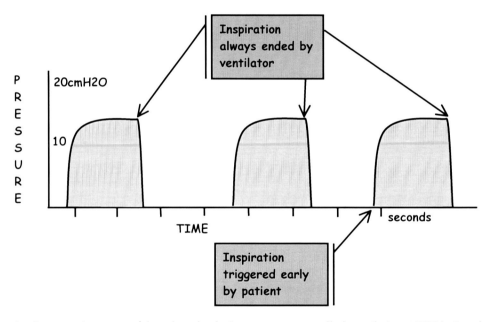

Figure 6.4 Pressure-time trace of three breaths during pressure-controlled ventilation: NIPPV. Breaths are usually initiated by the ventilator. They are all the same length, even if the patient triggers a breath.

**Terminology**

**Ventilator cycling: time or flow?**

In NIPPV, the beginning and end of each breath happens at a pre-determined time. This is called time-cycling. In BIPAP, the beginning and end of each breath is determined by changes in flow, so this is a flow-cycled mode. Time-cycling may kick in if the patient's rate drops too low.

## Summary

- Pressure support provides a positive pressure in time with the patient's own breathing cycle to help them breathe in.
- Bi-level pressure support (BIPAP) is pressure support with expiratory pressure added.
- The expiratory pressure is called EPAP.
- NIPPV is a pressure-control mode.
- BIPAP is flow-cycled, NIPPV is time-cycled.

# 7
# Circuits

---

## Learning points:

By the end of this chapter you should be able to:

- Put together a BIPAP circuit.

- Describe why rebreathing would occur if the expiratory port is blocked.

- Say why a bacterial filter should be placed over the ventilator outlet.

- Demonstrate how you would set up BIPAP.

- *Put together a NIPPV circuit.*

- *Demonstrate how you would set up NIPPV.*

- *Explain the consequences of transposing the exhalation valve and pressure sensing tubes of a NIPPV circuit.*

## Keywords:

Rebreathing.

---

## Circuits for BIPAP

A ventilator circuit needs to deliver air from the ventilator to the patient.  We could do this by using a length of standard 22mm tubing.   The problem with a simple tube is that the patient breathes out into the tubing, and then breathes the same "stale" air back in again.  You can try this for yourself just by breathing in and out of a length of tube – within a few breaths you start to feel pretty uncomfortable.  This is because you are breathing back in air which you have breathed out, which is low in oxygen but high in $CO_2$.  This is called rebreathing, which would be inevitable if we just connected a patient to their ventilator with a length of tubing.  We need to find a way of getting the stale air the patient has already breathed once out of the tubing before they take the next breath in.

## The expiratory port

The expiratory port is a small hole in the circuit, near to the mask. When the ventilator is pushing air into the patient, there is some leakage through this hole, but the ventilator is easily able to adjust for this:

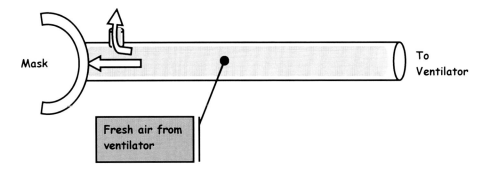

Figure 7.1 During inspiration, there is some leakage of air out through the expiratory port.

When the patient breathes out, the hole isn't big enough for all the exhaled air to pass through - some of the exhaled air goes down the main tube:

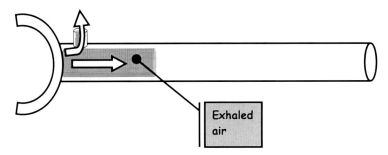

Figure 7.2 Exhaled air goes out of the expiratory port, and back up the ventilator tubing.

Later, as the flow from the patient tails off, the positive pressure in the circuit (EPAP) pushes the exhaled air back down the tube and out of the leakage hole:

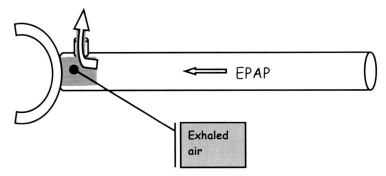

Figure 7.3 EPAP forces the exhaled air back down the ventilator tubing and out of the expiratory port.

Because the leak hole is fairly small, the ventilator can still sense when the patient wants to breathe in, so you don't need an additional tube to sense pressure at the mask. There is nothing special about the hole in the tube. It needs to be about 5mm in diameter - too small and the flow isn't enough to blow out exhaled air; if it is too big, there will be so much flow that the ventilator may struggle to get enough pressure to the patient. Your circuits will probably already come with an expiratory port, or you can attach a connector with a side hole - make sure no-one connects anything (such as oxygen tubing) to the hole inadvertently.

> **Key points**
>
> In BIPAP there is a small hole, or exhalation port, in the circuit near the mask to vent out exhaled air.

Purpose-made exhalation ports come in various degrees of sophistication, but the more complex they are the more expensive. If the mask you are using has access ports on it, you can open these up as the exhalation ports – provided the holes are big enough, this can be the best option for blowing out $CO_2$ because the holes are so close to the patient. If your patient's blood gases are not improving on BIPAP, always check that the expiratory port is not blocked. Finally, don't mistake the flow of air out through the expiratory port with a mask leak.

**Filters**

This circuit will be used on only one patient and then discarded, so cleaning the circuit isn't an issue. We'll come back to infection control later, but at this point we do need to put a bacterial filter at the ventilator end of the circuit. Since air is always blowing one way down the tubing, bacteria can't get much more than about 10cm upstream from the exhalation port. However, if some water condenses in the circuit or if the patient coughs some sputum into the tubing, it is possible for these liquids to run back into the ventilator by gravity if the other end of the circuit is higher. The inside of a ventilator is very difficult to sterilise, so as a precaution let's put a filter in to protect it. Make sure you use a simple (thin) bacterial filter, not a heat and moisture exchanger (HME) which would increase the resistance to flow, particularly when wet.

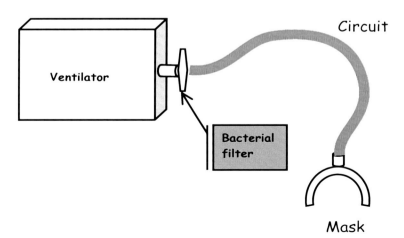

**Figure 7.4** A bacterial filter is placed on the ventilator outlet, to prevent the inside becoming contaminated.

**Start a patient with acute respiratory failure on BIPAP**

- Choose a mask.
- Get the right straps to hold it in place.
- Set up the circuit.
- Turn the ventilator on.
- Wait for any ventilator self-calibration or other set-up procedures to complete .
- If there is a choice of mode on the ventilator, choose bi-level pressure support or BIPAP.
- If the ventilator has an option with a back-up rate (eg assist/control) then choose that mode and set it to 12 breaths per minute*.
- Set the IPAP to 12cmH$_2$O.
- Set the EPAP to 5cmH$_2$O.
- Hold the mask on the patient, and ask them to breathe in and out of the mask so they get used to the sensation of the pressure from the ventilator.
- When they are settled, strap the mask in place.
- Watch for a few minutes.
- Check the oxygen saturation: if it less than 88%, put an oxygen connector in the circuit and start 1 L/min of oxygen, or set the oxygen concentration on the ventilator to 28% if you have this facility.*
- Set up appropriate monitoring.*
- Write down the ventilator settings and oxygen flow rate.
- Decide when you are going to re-evaluate (eg with a blood gas in one hour).*
- After discussion with all appropriate people, write down whether the patient is to be intubated if they deteriorate.*

If you felt comfortable doing this, you will be able to do it independently after a few more times. The steps marked with a * will make more sense in due course, but it will be easier to understand them if you have already done some basic NIV. If any of the steps not marked with a * are causing you concern, then go back a stage and re-read the relevant section.

## Circuits for NIPPV

NIPPV ventilators have a different way of preventing rebreathing. There is an exhalation valve near the mask which is closed when the ventilator is pushing air into the patient, so that the air doesn't escape through the valve rather than getting to the patient. It opens during expiration to let the air escape.

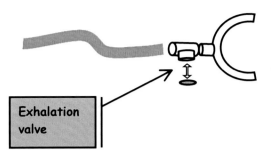

**Figure 7.5** NIPPV exhalation valve between the circuit tubing and the mask

You need an additional small tube to pressurize the valve to close it. When the valve is open during expiration, it is impossible for the ventilator to detect the negative pressure (or flow) which would indicate that the patient wants to trigger a breath; usually a third tube is needed to measure the pressure at the mask:

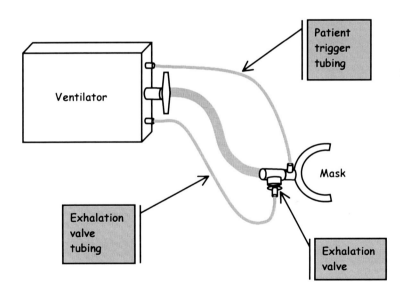

**Figure 7.6** Additional small-bore tubes to close the exhalation valve and to sense airway pressure

Clearly there is the possibility of these tubes becoming mixed up, so always check they are connected the right way round. You will know if they are the wrong way round because lots of air will be whooshing out of the expiratory valve during inspiration. Very occasionally the diaphragm in the valve may split or become folded – you can dismantle the valve to check this, or just change the circuit.

**Start a patient with chronic respiratory failure on NIPPV**

- Choose a mask.
- Get the right straps to hold it in place.
- Set up the circuit.
- Turn the ventilator on.
- Count the patient's spontaneous respiratory rate.
- Set the ventilator rate to the spontaneous rate.
- Adjust the timing of the ventilator so that the inspiration and expiration are approximately the same as the patient's own spontaneous breaths.
- Set the IPAP to 20cmH$_2$O.
- Hold the mask on the patient, and ask them to breathe in and out of the mask so they get used to the sensation of the pressure from the ventilator.
- When they have grown accustomed to NIV, strap the mask in place.
- Watch for a few minutes.
- Adjust the mask to minimize leaks.
- Adjust the pressure up or down, within the range 15-30cmH$_2$O, to the lowest level that gives good chest expansion.
- See if the patient feels comfortable with a slightly slower respiratory rate.
- Write down the ventilator settings.

## Infection control

In acute respiratory failure, circuits should be used on one patient only. There is no need to change the circuit daily - as with masks, circuits that look clean are generally fine from a microbiological point of view. For long-term NIV at home, circuits should be washed once a week in warm soapy water - or in a dish washer – and hung up to dry thoroughly. Some ventilators have the clever option of allowing you to blow air down the circuit to dry it. There is usually no need to change the circuit more frequently than once every few weeks.

If the exhalation port or valve is placed at the ventilator end of the circuit rather than the mask end, the patient will inevitably re-breathe only exhaled air. This is an easy mistake to make – always check the circuit.

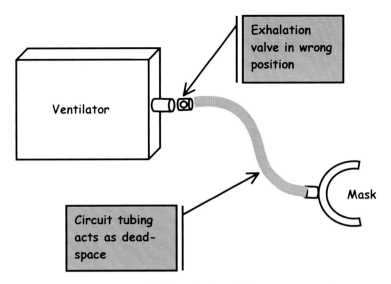

**Figure** 7.7 If the circuit is assembled with the exhalation port or valve at the wrong end, re-breathing is inevitable.

## Summary

- The circuit for BIPAP is a large tube, with a small hole near the patient end, out of which exhaled air escapes.
- A bacterial filter at the other end stops the ventilator from becoming contaminated.
- Circuits for NIPPV have an exhalation valve, which is closed during inspiration by pressure supplied through a separate small bore tube.
- In NIPPV a third tube is used to detect airway pressure, to allow the patient to trigger the ventilator.
- In NIPPV set the ventilator so that the timing is the same as the patient's own breathing.
- Use higher IPAP pressures initially for NIPPV than you would for BIPAP.

# 8

# Chronic Obstructive Pulmonary Disease

---

**Learning points:**

By the end of this chapter you should be able to:

- Decide when to start a patient with COPD on NIV.

- Connect oxygen or a nebulizer to NIV.

- *Explain why supplementary oxygen may be harmful in COPD.*

- *Discuss which COPD patients might benefit from long-term NIV.*

---

Patients who need NIV acutely can be split into three groups:

A. Those with common diseases such as COPD or left ventricular failure (LVF) who present with acute hypercapnic respiratory failure and need NIV for a few hours or days during the acute illness.  Their pH level will be low.

B. Those with fairly normal lungs who slip into hypercapnic respiratory failure because their breathing muscles give up or their central respiratory drive is poor (ventilatory pump failure).  Many of these patients will need long term NIV at home.  Sometimes you get warning that trouble is brewing and can start NIV electively, but quite often there is a crisis and NIV is started acutely

C. The rest.

In this chapter we'll look at the commonest situation in which NIV is needed – an acute exacerbation of COPD.

## Which COPD patients?

NIV is not indicated in an acute exacerbation of COPD if the patient does not have a respiratory acidosis.  Perhaps the commonest mistake in NIV is to use it in a patient with COPD whose pH level is greater than 7.35.  If the patient does become acidotic, NIV can be used much earlier than intubation in the course of the exacerbation to break the downward spiral into increasingly severe acidosis.

**Key points**

In acute exacerbations of COPD, only use NIV in patients with a respiratory acidosis (pH <7.35)

Before you have to decide whether or not to use NIV, you will usually have time to administer drug therapy - such as nebulized bronchodilators - and set up properly controlled oxygen therapy. After an hour or so, if things are not improving then it is time for NIV. By this time you should have had a chance to move the patient to HDU, or a similar area where NIV is used regularly. Some patients are so sick that you should intubate them and ventilate them invasively: these patients are usually more acidotic. Severe acidosis in itself does not preclude a trial of NIV if it is safe to do so; you may have to start NIV sooner - in the ED or AMU - but the patient needs to be transferred to ICU as soon as possible.

Thin COPD patients don't tend to do terribly well on NIV, but it is still worth a trial. The reason for this is not clear, but my interpretation is that these thin patients are "pink puffers" with high respiratory drives who are not normally hypercapnic; the fact they have slipped into type 2 respiratory failure indicates they have run out of lung and are nearing the end of their life.

## What ventilator settings?

As we've already mentioned, BIPAP is the best mode for COPD. The starting pressures I recommend are an IPAP of $12cmH_2O$ and an EPAP of $5cmH_2O$. You may need to push up the IPAP slowly towards $20cmH_2O$ during the course of the next few hours depending on the response, but most COPD patients will be intolerant of NIV if you start at $20cmH_2O$. To achieve effective ventilation you may even need to go up to $30cmH_2O$, but in COPD you should start fairly low and build the IPAP up. We'll see in the chapter on triggering why it may be necessary to increase the EPAP slightly, but not above $10cmH_2O$. Set the back-up rate to about 10 breaths per minute, with an inspiratory:expiratory ratio of 1:3 for these breaths, to leave the patient plenty of time to breathe out - more of this in the chapter on I:E ratios.

## Oxygen

If the oxygen saturation is below 88% once the patient is established on NIV, then add supplemental oxygen, starting at 1 L/min and increasing until the saturation runs between 88 and 92%. The patient gets better through a combination of their own respiratory effort and NIV. If you give too much oxygen they will stop breathing, leaving NIV to provide all the ventilation, which may not be enough. In a significant proportion of COPD admissions the acidosis is made worse by administration of high concentrations of oxygen on the journey in to hospital.

**Practical Tip**

**Oxygen and nebulizers during NIV**

The best place to add oxygen or nebulized drugs to a NIV circuit is just by the exhale port or valve, on the ventilator side. This allows the ventilator tubing to act as a reservoir for the oxygen or bronchodilators during expiration.

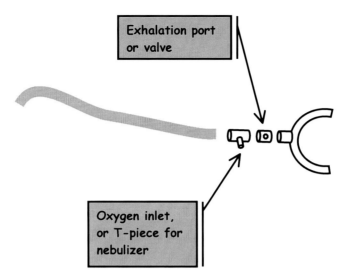

**Figure 8.1** Connect oxygen or a nebulizer to a NIV circuit on the ventilator side
(as opposed to the patient side) of the expiratory port or valve.

## How long for?

If after one hour of NIV the acidosis is not improving, you should consider abandoning NIV and intubating the patient. You may have time to adjust the ventilator settings (mainly by increasing the IPAP) and re-assess after another hour or so, but if there has been no improvement after 4 hours then NIV is probably not doing any good and should be stopped. Aim for NIV most of the time for the first 24 hours, accepting that in practice the patient will only spend about 15 hours on the ventilator by the time they have had breaks for nebulizers, meals etc. The next day you can plan longer breaks, but they will probably still use NIV overnight. By the day after that, the patient will normally be better and probably refusing to use NIV anyway.

*Key points*

It will usually be apparent after about an hour of NIV whether or not it is going to work in acute respiratory failure.

## Long term

There are trials in progress to see whether NIV using high inflation pressures, titrated to correct nocturnal hypoventilation, will benefit a wider group of patients with COPD in the longer term. For the moment, here are some reasons why you might want to use NIV at home in COPD:

· **Recurrent episodes of respiratory acidosis**

Longer-term NIV is needed in only a small proportion of patients with COPD. If the patient has had more than three exacerbations requiring NIV within the last six months (and has tolerated

NIV well), then you should consider leaving them on it at night at home indefinitely. These patients are usually obese with poor respiratory drive, and probably overlap with the obesity-hypoventilation syndrome. Ask the patient – success is more likely if they are keen to use NIV and feel it does them some good.

· **Nocturnal hypoventilation with sleep disturbance**

We all have a slightly higher $PaCO_2$ at night than during the day, reflecting lower alveolar ventilation during sleep. Patients with hypercapnia will always be worse during sleep. If they wake up frequently during the night, they can experience excessive sleepiness during the daytime. A trial of NIV is warranted in these patients to see if it improves their sleepiness. After a month or so, let the patient decide if they want to continue with it.

· **Long term oxygen**

Sometimes NIV is the only way you can establish a patient with COPD on long-term oxygen therapy without inducing dangerous hypercapnia. We use the lowest $FiO_2$ which gets the $PaO_2$ above 8kPa - if this causes the $PaCO_2$ to rise above 10kPa then it is probably safer to use NIV (in combination with oxygen).

*Physiology*

**Work of breathing**

To get air into the lungs, the inspiratory muscles use energy. This energy is needed to overcome two different factors – the "elastic" tendency of the lungs to collapse like a balloon, and the "resistance" to flow of air down the airways.

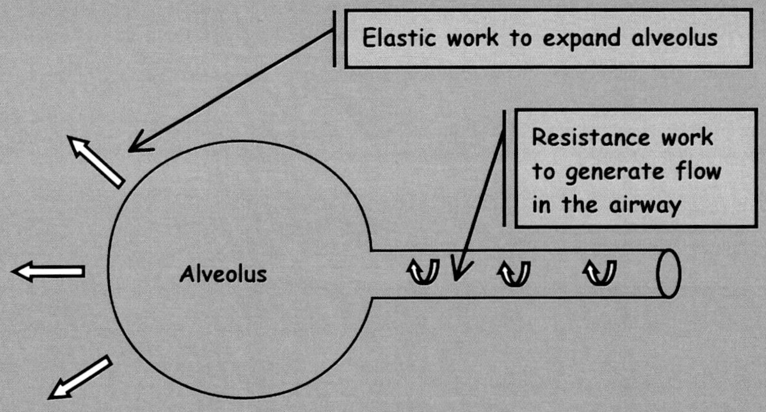

**Figure 8.2** The work of breathing.

The work of breathing can be thought of as the load on the muscles. Like any other muscle, the breathing muscles have a limited capacity to do work. We'll come back to the concept of load versus capacity later.

## Summary

- In acute exacerbations of COPD, NIV helps patients with an acute respiratory acidosis (pH <7.35)

- If you need to add oxygen or a nebulizer, position it near the exhalation port, but on the ventilator rather than the patient side.

- Very few patients with COPD need NIV long-term

# 9

# Inspiratory Pressure

---

## Learning points

By the end of this chapter you should be able to:

- Decide when to increase IPAP.

- *Define span.*

- *Describe rise time and when to reduce it.*

- *Explain how compliance affects NIV.*


## Keywords:

Span, Rise time.

---

We have noted already that when you blow air into a patient's lungs with a ventilator, the harder you blow (ie the more IPAP) the more air you will get in. Earlier, when we started a patient on BIPAP we used 12cmH$_2$O for the IPAP, but for NIPPV we selected 20cmH$_2$O. The range of IPAP we have to play with is between 10 and 30cmH$_2$O. Here are a few points about IPAP:

- Higher pressures produce a higher Vt, so if your patient gets used to NIV but their blood gases don't improve, try increasing the pressure.

- Increasing IPAP may also increase leaks.

- If you increase IPAP (or EPAP) you will blow more oxygen out of the expiratory port - to keep the same FiO$_2$, you may need to increase the oxygen flow rate.

- You won't be able to get inspiratory pressures much above 30cmH$_2$O because the mask blows off the face.

- An IPAP of less than 10cmH$_2$O provides very little assistance to ventilation.

If you want to get more air into the lungs, increase the IPAP

## IPAP and Span

Span is a term you may come across which is used for the difference between IPAP and EPAP. Vt depends on this difference.

With BIPAP we often use an EPAP of $5cmH_2O$; the difference between this and an IPAP of 15 $cmH_2O$ is $10cmH_2O$. Increase the EPAP to $10cmH_2O$ and the difference between this and the IPAP – "span" – is only $5cmH_2O$. You may hear the terms "low span" and "high span" used in ICU.

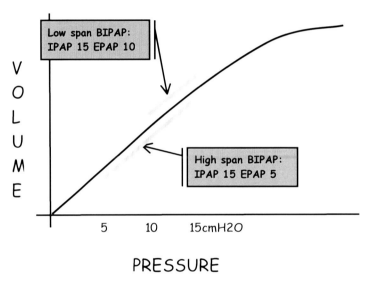

**Figure 9.1** Pressure-volume curve, showing effect of pressure on tidal volumes with BIPAP.

When someone tells you that a patient is on BIPAP of "10 over 5", check whether they mean an inspiratory pressure of 10 or $15cmH_2O$.

## Rise time

Some ventilators have the facility to adjust "rise time" (or "ramp"). Usually you won't have to worry about this, but now would be a good time just to explain what this means. When the ventilator triggers into inspiration, it takes a little while for it to reach the target IPAP, particularly if you are using higher pressures. So if the respiratory rate is very fast the patient won't get the IPAP you intended. One way of correcting this problem is to shorten the rise time, if this facility is available on your ventilator.

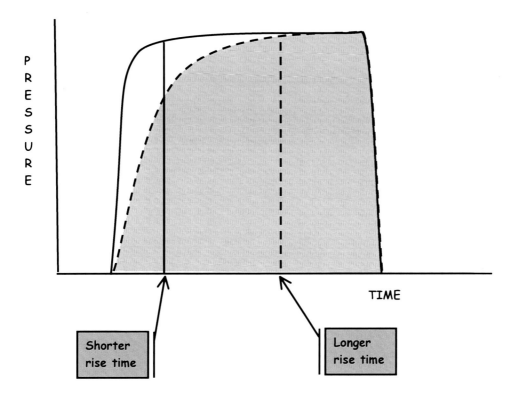

**Figure 9.2** Shorter and longer rise times. The target IPAP is reached much sooner with a shorter rise time.

In practice, you don't usually need to worry about rise time, except in patients with very high respiratory drive who are breathing very fast. It is worth just looking at the pressure indicator on the ventilator (on the graphical display or other indicator) to check that the target pressure is being reached by the end of inspiration. Shortening the rise time may help with this.

## Compliance

In the last chapter we mentioned the elastic work required to inflate the lungs. Another word for elasticity is "compliance". Very stiff lungs (for example in fibrotic lung disease) are not very compliant, and you need to use more pressure. In normal subjects, a pressure of about 10cmH$_2$O is required to get one litre of air into the lungs.

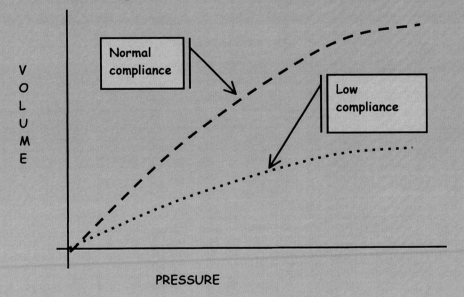

**Figure 9.3** Pressure-volume curves of the lung. When compliance is low, the increase in volume is much less as pressure increases.

In practice, it is quite difficult to measure lung compliance – you need an oesophageal balloon to get an estimate of the pleural pressure – and the normal values are not well defined.

## Summary

- More IPAP means more ventilation.
- In BIPAP, increasing EPAP will reduce ventilation by reducing span.
- Check that the patient is actually getting the pressure you have set.
- Occasionally you may need to shorten the rise time (ramp) in a very breathless patient.

# 10

# Assist/Control or Spontaneous/Timed

## Learning points

By the end of this chapter you should be able to:

- Outline the difference between assist and control (or spontaneous and timed) modes.
- Choose a back-up rate.
- *Describe why we use "Assist/Control" for most NIV applications.*

## Keywords

Assist, Control.

NIV ventilators sometimes have an option to choose "assist" or "assist/control" mode. Other options you may come across are "spontaneous" and "timed". Most of the ventilators you are likely to use will operate by default in a safe assist/control mode anyway, but if you have the option to choose and want to understand the difference then read on.

## Ventilatory Assistance

Assistance to breathing is exactly the principle we discussed under pressure support, whereby each breath is triggered by the patient. If the patient doesn't breathe, nothing happens. This mode is called "assist", "spontaneous" or both - "assisted spontaneous breathing (ASB)".

## Ventilatory Control

In control mode, the ventilator decides when each breath happens, according to the rate it has been set at.

## Assist/Control

You will probably have worked out that assist/control is assist with a back-up rate to kick in if the patient stops breathing. In some ventilators the back-up rate can be set, in others it is factory set. Ten or twelve breaths per minute will do as a back-up rate for most patients.

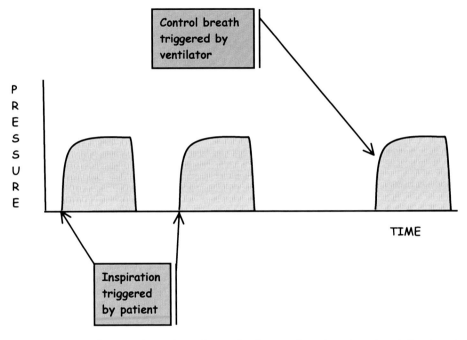

**Figure 10.1** Assist-control NIV. The patient triggers the first two breaths; when they fail to breathe faster than the back-up rate, the ventilator delivers a control breath.

## Summary

- Assist/control is the usual mode in which NIV is used.
- If the patient stops breathing, the ventilator continues to ventilate at a back-up rate.
- The back-up rate should be set at about 10-12 breaths per minute.

# 11

# Non-invasive or Invasive?

## Learning points:

By the end of this chapter you should be able to:

- Decide which patients should be intubated straight away rather than managed with NIV.
- Discuss how you would decide whether or not to proceed to intubation if your patient does not improve on NIV.
- *Explain how you would go about withdrawing NIV from a patient.*

## Keywords

Aspiration.

We try to avoid intubating patients if we possibly can:

- The need for sedation means that getting back to spontaneous breathing may be a problem.
- The patient cannot eat, so artificial feeding will be needed.
- Hospital—acquired pneumonia is a real worry.
- Other complications may develop in ICU.
- ICU beds are scarce.

Nevertheless, there are some patients for whom intubation is a better option than NIV right from the start. There are others who may not do well on NIV and we need to revert to intubation in order to ventilate them properly. On the other hand, it is inappropriate to intubate if there is no possibility of the patient surviving. How do we identify those who are not going to do well?

# Immediate intubation rather than NIV

Intubation is usually better than NIV for patients with any of the following:

- Impaired conscious level (GCS <7).
- Multi-organ failure.
- Severe hypoxia.
- Respiratory arrest.
- Total ventilator dependence.
- Fixed upper airway obstruction.
- Facial burns/trauma.
- Head trauma/CSF leaks.
- Sinus/middle ear infection.
- Recent oesophageal/gastric surgery.
- Copious sputum production.

Most of the reasons are self-explanatory, but let's look at a few critical points in more detail.

## Airway protection

If a patient on NIV vomits, there is a  risk that they may inhale the vomit into their lungs.  This is a big  worry in an unconscious patient.  If you vomit, you contract your laryngeal muscles to close your vocal cords tight shut.  You don't take a breath in until you have cleared all the vomit from your throat.  If anything does go down the wrong way into your lungs, you cough and splutter until it comes out again.  An unconscious patient on NIV may vomit or regurgitate gastric contents into their pharynx.  When the ventilator applies a positive pressure, gastric contents are pushed down into the lungs.  The result is aspiration pneumonia. Some conscious patients with poor laryngeal  muscle function, for example after a stroke or in motor neurone disease, may also be unable to protect their airway from aspiration during NIV.

> **Key points**
>
> In NIV the airway is not protected against aspiration.

## Safe ventilation

On ICU, a ventilated patient has their endotracheal or tracheostomy tube secured in place with ties (or sometimes stitches in the case of a tracheostomy tube).   The patient is usually pretty immobile, and so the chances of the ventilator becoming disconnected are low.  In contrast, a patient on NIV is conscious and able to move their head; their ventilator is attached by some straps fastened with Velcro, and the mask can become displaced. It the patient is unable to breathe spontaneously at all, then disconnection could be disastrous.

## Effective ventilation

- With invasive ventilation, inflation pressures up to 60cmH$_2$O are sometimes used to ventilate patients with very stiff lungs or tight airways. With NIV, pressures much above 30cmH$_2$O cause the mask to blow off the face of the patient, resulting in intolerable leaks. This is good in that barotrauma (damage caused by high inflation pressures) to the lung is not going to be a problem, but it does mean that some patients will need to be intubated in order to get higher inflation pressures.

- With many (but not all) NIV ventilators, it is impossible to get the inspired oxygen concentration above 40%. If the patient has such a severe problem with gas exchange that they need more oxygen than this, they will need to be intubated.

- During NIV, the patient is awake and breathing with their own rhythm, or something pretty close. When they are sedated and intubated you have much more scope to play around with the timing of respiration in order to try and improve gas exchange.

## Secretions

Every time a patient wants to cough out secretions from their lungs, they need to take off their mask. This is fine if it only happens every few minutes, but if they have a very productive cough – for example in bronchiectasis – then they will spend all the time taking the mask on and off and derive no benefit from the ventilator. Intubation will probably be a better option if the patient is coughing up sputum most of the time.

> **Key points**
>
> Intubate the patient on the basis of their clinical condition, taking into account their arterial blood gas values - not on the blood gas values alone.

## NIV for patients who are not for intubation

If you decide in advance that intubation is not an option, there is nothing to stop you trying NIV in patients with any of the contraindications listed at the beginning of the chapter, for example an unconscious patient or someone with severe hypoxia. If you are aware of the potential complications you can take measures to minimise the risk.

> **Practical Tip**
>
> In a patient who is not for intubation, beware of persevering with NIV for too long, past the point where there is any hope of the patient surviving.

**Ventilate an unconscious patient using NIV**

*   Keep the patient propped up in bed as high as you can.
*   Use a full face mask.
*   Pass a nasogastric tube first.
*   Aspirate the nasogastric tube regularly to keep the stomach empty.
*   Start the patient on drugs to reduce gastric acidity, to minimise the chemical damage to the lungs if they do aspirate.
*   Aspirate pharyngeal secretions regularly.

## Intubation when NIV fails

A patient may deteriorate on NIV, and you have to decide whether to intubate or not. There are two crucial questions to ask:

### Has it been possible to establish the patient on NIV?

If the patient has failed to settle on NIV for some reason, for example because they cannot tolerate a mask, then they have not really had a trial of assisted ventilation. You need a different interface between the patient and the ventilator – an endotracheal tube – to see if ventilation is going to work. On the other hand you may have settled the patient onto NIV fairly quickly, then increased the IPAP to 20cmH$_2$O or so and added supplementary oxygen. If they fail to improve at this point then it is failure of assisted ventilation, rather than failure of NIV. Changing the interface to an endotracheal tube is going to make much less difference than in the patient who couldn't tolerate a mask – the rewards of intubation are likely to be lower.

### Is the patient likely to survive intubation?

This is a difficult decision and there isn't much decent quality data on which to base it. The bottom line is that patients often do much better than expected, and if in doubt they should be intubated. In patients with an acute exacerbation of COPD, there are a few factors which are commonly used to identify patients who don't do well:

*   No clear reversible reason for deterioration.

*   Normal CXR. (No pneumonia or pneumothorax as a reversible cause for deterioration, implying that the patient has simply run out of functioning lung).

*   Presence of co-morbidities.

*   Poor exercise tolerance (housebound) prior to exacerbation.

## Summary

- Intubation is a better option for unconscious patients who are unable to protect their own airway.

- Careful monitoring in HDU or ICU is mandatory if NIV is used in patients who are unable to do at least some breathing for themselves.

- Intubation is usually better than NIV for patients with severe hypoxia or multiple system failure.

- Don't delay intubation by tinkering around for too long with NIV in a severely ill patient.

# 12

# Left Ventricular Failure

---

## Learning points

By the end of this chapter you should be able to:

* Decide which patients with LVF need NIV.

* Set a patient with LVF up on NIV.

* *Say what to look for to make sure that NIV is working.*

* *Decide where to manage a patient with LVF on NIV.*

* *Discuss the use of NIV in chronic heart failure.*

---

Sometimes it can be difficult to decide whether acute breathlessness is COPD or LVF. The good news is that NIV works for both, although there has been quite of lot of debate about its use in heart failure. Some early trials used NIV without much else in the way of drug treatment, and in one of the first randomized studies the patients who were treated with NIV by chance had more severe myocardial ischaemia and not surprisingly did less well.

## Which patients?

Drug therapy is the mainstay of treatment of acute LVF, but if the patient is hypercapnic they will get better more quickly with BIPAP. NIV also reduces the intubation rate in hypercapnic patients. You could try CPAP first and move to BIPAP is this fails, but I think it is quite reasonable to go straight to BIPAP if the $PaCO_2$ is high.

### *Practical Tip*

Use CPAP for LVF if the $PaCO_2$ is normal or low, BIPAP if the $PaCO_2$ is high.

## What ventilator settings?

Use BIPAP starting with an IPAP of 10cmH$_2$O and an EPAP of 5cmH$_2$O. Depending on the patient's respiratory pattern, this is equivalent to using CPAP of about 7.5cmH$_2$O, which would be quite a reasonable starting level if we weren't using NIV.  Nudge both the IPAP and EPAP down 2cmH$_2$O if the patient's blood pressure does drop.  Increasing the IPAP to 15cmH$_2$O will help a persistently elevated PaCO$_2$, whereas increasing the EPAP to 7 or 8cmH$_2$O should improve oxygenation.  Set the back-up rate to about 10 breaths/min, with an inspiratory:expiratory ratio of 1:2.

## Where?

Start NIV early in LVF – you don't have as much time to play with as in COPD.  The patient will need ECG and saturation monitoring, so they really need to be on a coronary care unit, HDU or ICU as soon as possible.  The decision between CCU and HDU will depend on whether thrombolysis is needed, how likely serious cardiac dysrhythmias are and the NIV experience of CCU staff.

## How long for?

A few hours of NIV is often all that is necessary.  After this time, drug therapy will have kicked in and the patient will start to improve.

---

*How to do it*

**Transfer a patient on NIV**

- Check that the receiving clinical area is ready.

- Things tend to become dislodged during transfer – ensure all vascular lines, the NIV mask etc are secured in place.

- If the NIV ventilator does not have an internal battery, connect an external battery.

- Check that the batteries are fully charged.

- If the patient needs supplementary oxygen, change the supply to a cylinder.

- Secure the ventilator, battery and oxygen cylinder to the trolley or bed, in a position where they cannot fall onto the floor or onto the patient.

- Attach a battery-powered pulse oximeter to the patient.

- Take a resuscitation bag and mask with you.

- If the patient is for intubation if they deteriorate, take the appropriate equipment with you.

- Transfer the patient.

Most patients on NIV can manage spontaneous breathing for a few minutes: it is much easier to transfer a patient off NIV. Transferring unstable patients on NIV is risky – are you sure it would not be better to intubate them?

## NIV in chronic heart failure

Some patients with chronic heart failure have disturbed sleep, usually associated with Cheyne-Stoke's respiration. This is cyclical increase and decrease in Vt, so that sometimes the patient is hyperventilating and sometimes they stop breathing. Long-term NIV at home may help these patients. When we look at volume-controlled ventilation, we'll see how it is possible to use a ventilator which will follow the cyclical changes in Vt. We are still exploring the role of nocturnal NIV in chronic heart failure – the number of patients who benefit is likely to remain small, given that excessive daytime sleepiness (in contrast to fatigue) is an uncommon symptom in this condition.

*Physiology*

**Oxygen delivery**

We have talked already about $PaO_2$ and $SpO_2$. Remember that the oxygen content of blood is also dependent on the haemoglobin concentration: the number of mls of oxygen in each litre is given by the following equation:

$$SpO_2 \times Hb \times 13.4$$

The blood also needs to be transported to the peripheral tissues, so clearly cardiac output will be important. Cardiac output depends on the volume of blood leaving the heart with each beat (stroke volume) and the heart rate. Oxygen delivery can be calculated by:

$$Stroke\ volume \times heart\ rate \times SpO_2 \times Hb \times 13.4$$

The 13.4 value isn't important to remember, but bear the other factors in mind when you are trying to maximise oxygen delivery to the peripheral tissues in a patient with heart failure.

## Summary

- NIV is an effective treatment for LVF.

- Use it if the patient does not respond to initial drug therapy.

- Use BIPAP and keep the pressure fairly low.

- Don't forget to give drugs.

- Stop NIV as soon as the patient is better.

# 13

# Expiratory Pressure

## Learning points

By the end of this chapter you should be able to:

- Define EPAP.
- *Define the upper and lower limits you would normally use for EPAP.*
- *List the physiological effects of EPAP.*
- *Discuss the clinical situations in which it may be helpful to alter EPAP.*

## Keywords:

Expiratory positive airway pressure, Intrinsic positive end-expiratory pressure.

For most patients on BIPAP, an EPAP of 5cmH$_2$O will be fine. You don't need to adjust it very often. IPAP is much more important. As you become more conversant with NIV you may start to adjust the EPAP from time to time, but the range is pretty narrow and the benefits usually small. Many patients find EPAP a bit uncomfortable, and few will tolerate more than 10cmH$_2$O.

## Flushing CO$_2$ out of the circuit

We have seen how EPAP flushes exhaled air out of the expiratory port of the circuit, allowing us to use a single tube. If the patient settles well onto NIV and their chest seems to be expanding well in time with the ventilation but the PaCO$_2$ fails to fall, it is worth just thinking about increasing the EPAP a little in case re-breathing is occurring. The higher the EPAP the more flow there will be out of the expiratory port. Remember that increasing the EPAP will also flush oxygen out of the circuit. If you have a single-tube BIPAP circuit, don't reduce EPAP below 3cmH$_2$O.

## Upper airway patency

EPAP keeps the upper airway open, just as CPAP does in the treatment of obstructive sleep apnoea. Although IPAP would open the airway in due course anyway, the fact that it is held open by EPAP allows the ventilator to sense when the patient wants to take the next breath in. If a very obese patient appears to be trying to take a breath in, but the ventilator is not triggering, think about upper airway obstruction – try increasing the EPAP to 10cmH$_2$O.

## Oxygenation

EPAP increases lung volume, which is good if there is a problem with oxygenation on account of lung collapse (atelectasis) in the lower parts of the lung. There is a downside to increasing lung volume, in that you may over-inflate the more distensible parts of the lung. The blood vessels in over-inflated areas of lung are stretched and thin, so you may divert blood towards the stiffer parts of the lung which can't over-inflate – these may well be areas of diseased lung which don't exchange gas very well.

## Ventilation

In type 1 respiratory failure, we may choose to use an EPAP of up to 10cmH$_2$O. You may remember from the chapter on IPAP that this reduces the difference between IPAP and EPAP, so the tidal volume will be less – keep an eye on the PaCO$_2$.

Over-inflation is particularly bad for COPD patients, putting their respiratory muscles at even more of a mechanical disadvantage than they are already.

## Cardiac output

EPAP increases the pressure inside the chest, and this may impede the return of venous blood from the periphery – if the mean intrathoracic pressure is high, the pressure needed to push the blood back into heart is higher. The result of this is that cardiac output may fall. If there is a fall in blood pressure on BIPAP, reduce both the IPAP and EPAP and consider administering intravenous fluids.

## Intrinsic PEEP

Intrinsic PEEP (PEEPi or "autopeep" as it is sometimes called) is a particular feature of patients with airflow obstruction such as COPD. It is a difficult concept to explain, not made any easier by the difficulty of measuring it – you would need an oesophageal pressure probe or balloon. The "intrinsic" bit comes from ICU, where "extrinsic" PEEP (positive end-expiratory pressure) is used as another term for EPAP.

So, let's ignore the "PEEP" bit, forget about the "intrinsic" bit and concentrate on why PEEPi makes it hard work for COPD patients to trigger inspiration during NIV.

If you take a breath in and then relax all your respiratory and upper airway muscles, the air in your lungs flows out quickly, usually much less than one second. When you contract your inspiratory muscles, flow starts straight away, and if you were connected to an NIV ventilator, inspiration would be triggered immediately.

In a patient with narrow airways, it could take up to 30 seconds for the lungs to empty completely. Clearly a patient with COPD is not going to take one breath every minute, they cannot breathe that slowly, so the result is that they have not fully exhaled when they start to take the next breath in.

Let's suppose that there is still a litre of air in the lungs left to exhale when they have to take another breath in. The inspiratory muscles have to contract as if they were inhaling this litre before they get up to the position where the lungs have stopped because of the trapped air. Only then does flow start so the ventilator can trigger. The pressure that the inspiratory muscles have to generate before there is any airflow is equivalent to PEEPi.

You can use EPAP to help the patient overcome PEEPi. Increasing the EPAP means that the patient will start from a point much nearer the lung volume they are trapped at, so they don't need to make such a big effort to get some flow and trigger the ventilator:

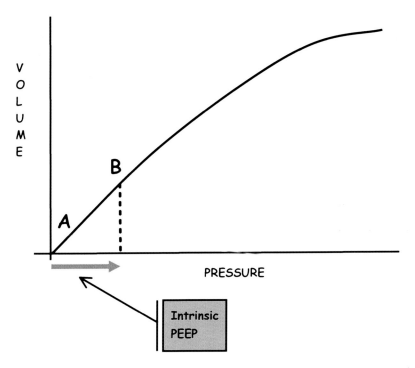

**Figure 13.1** Intrinsic PEEP. At the end of expiration, a normal person would be at point A; when they generate pressure to inflate their lungs, by using their inspiratory muscles, volume starts to increase straight away – if they were on NIV, this change in volume (flow) would be sensed by the ventilator which would immediately assist the breath. In severe COPD, airway collapse means that at the end of expiration the patient has so much air trapped in their lung that they are at point B; when they contract their inspiratory muscles, there will be no change in lung volume until they have generated a pressure equivalent to being at point B – only then is there any flow to tell the ventilator that they want to take a breath in.

## Why do airways collapse in expiration?

If you think of a fire-fighter's hose (the thin collapsible sort you can roll up flat), the pressure at the tap end is high (let's call this pressure A), and at the end the water comes out is zero (or atmospheric). When there is water flowing down the hose, pressure falls from A to zero along the length of the hose because of the resistance to flow. The pressure in an airway behaves in the same way:

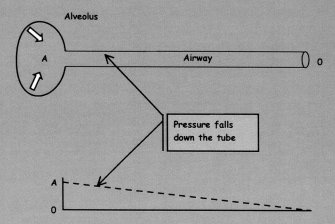

Imagine putting the tap and the hose inside a big tank, leaving the end of the hose sticking out, and pressurising the tank – let's call this pressure B. The "driving pressure" at the tap end of the hose is now the tap pressure plus the pressure inside the tank. The pressure at the hose outlet is still zero, so the pressure inside the hose must fall steadily from A+B to zero as we move from the tap to the open end. The pressure outside the hose is B all the way along its length, because it is inside the tank. At some point along the length of the hose, as pressure falls from A+B to zero, this pressure will become less than B and the hose will collapse:

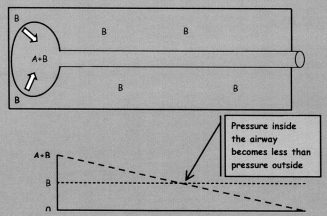

In the lungs, A is the elastic recoil of the alveoli and B is the expiratory pressure we generate with our expiratory muscles. Usually A is sufficiently high that the pressure inside the hose doesn't fall from A+B to B until we reach the large airways, which are splinted open by cartilage and don't collapse. If A is very low, because of emphysema, then the pressure inside the airways falls to B very quickly and the airways collapse.

## Summary

- EPAP flushes $CO_2$ out of the BIPAP circuit.
- Upper airway patency is maintained.
- Lung volume is increased.
- Cardiac output may decrease.
- EPAP helps overcome PEEPi.

# 14
# Monitoring

## Learning points

By the end of this chapter you should be able to:

- Set up monitoring for a patient with acute respiratory failure on NIV.
- Explain the parameters displayed on the ventilator panel.
- *Explain the relationship between oxygen saturation and alveolar ventilation.*

Monitoring is essential when you are looking after someone in acute respiratory failure, more so than when you are starting NIV electively in chronic hypercapnic respiratory failure.

## Look at the patient

When you have started a patient on NIV, the most important thing to do is look at them from the bedside:

- Is their chest moving?
- Are they still using their accessory muscles?
- How comfortable do they look?

Look at the patient first, then look at the ventilator: if the patient is not synchronising with the ventilator, then the numbers shown on the ventilator may be misleading.

## Basic monitoring

The next thing to do when assessing how a patient is doing on NIV is to look at simple physiological variables:

- Respiratory rate.
- Pulse rate.
- Blood pressure.
- $SpO_2$.

## Respiratory rate

In many clinical situations a fast respiratory rate is an important indicator that the patient is very unwell.  As they improve, the respiratory rate will gradually fall back to normal.  This is true when NIV is used to treat acute respiratory failure, provided the patient is triggering the ventilator (as is usually the case with BIPAP, unless the back-up rate is set too high)

### Pulse rate

Tachycardia is also common in acute respiratory failure, and a fall in pulse rate back towards normal when NIV is started is also a reassuring indicator that the patient is improving. Bradycardia is worrying, and implies an impending crisis (unless there is an obvious explanation such as beta-blockade).

### Blood pressure

The blood pressure response to NIV is less predictable.   If the patient is anxious or extremely unwell, they may be hypertensive initially and fall to more normal levels when they are settled on NIV.  Conversely, the blood pressure may be low initially in a patient who is very hypoxic and hypercapnic, and may improve as NIV improves their gas exchange.  NIV creates a positive pressure within the thorax, which may impair venous return to the heart and thus lower the blood pressure.  This is uncommon, but you may need to reduce the IPAP and EPAP.

### Oxygen saturation

A patient with acute respiratory  failure is likely to have their oxygen saturation monitored using a pulse oximeter and finger probe.  This is extremely useful when the patient is breathing air.  Aim for an $SpO_2$ of 88-92%.  Much higher than this and you run the risk of suppressing the patient's own respiratory drive if there is any suggestion that respiratory failure is chronic. NIV is a form of assisted ventilation – it works best when assisting the patient's own breathing, particularly when you are using BIPAP in the acute setting.

### SpO$_2$ and hypercapnia when breathing supplementary oxygen

The alveolar air equation tells us about the partial pressure of oxygen in the alveoli. The abbreviation for this is PAO$_2$, with a capital A for alveolar:

$$PAO_2 = (FiO_2 \times 94) - (1.25 \times PaCO_2)$$

This is in kPa – change the 94 to 713 if you are using mmHg. According to this equation, if the PaCO$_2$ rises, then PAO$_2$ must fall. If the patient is breathing air, then they will desaturate and you will be alerted by the alarm on an oximeter.

If the patient is breathing supplementary oxygen, the PAO$_2$ will remain high when the PaCO$_2$ rises, so an oximeter will not alert you to hypercapnia. The reason for this is apparent if you look at the first part of the equation: FiO$_2$ x 94. Atmospheric pressure is 100kPa, but we have to take off about 6kPa to account for water vapour, since the alveolar air is fully humidified. You may remember that FiO$_2$ is the fraction of inspired oxygen – 0.21 for air. 0.21 x 94 gives 20 for the first part of the equation. On 60% oxygen, this becomes 56 (0.6 x 94), so the PaCO$_2$ would have to rise to impossible levels before the PAO$_2$ fell to the levels associated with desaturation. PaO$_2$ is always slightly lower than PAO$_2$, and desaturation below 90% occurs at around 8kPa.

## Blood gases

You will need to check blood gases after about an hour of NIV, and an hour after any change in settings. If the patient is really sick and in ICU or HDU, you may choose to insert an arterial line. It takes a while for blood gas values to improve, and the PaCO$_2$ may lag behind the pH. Carbon dioxide tension can be monitored continuously using a transcutaneous electrode. The accuracy of the readings is improved if an arterial sample is taken initially to assess the arterial-transcutaneous difference. End-tidal carbon dioxide tensions can be used to estimate PaCO$_2$, but should be used with caution in patients with abnormal lungs (ie most NIV patients).

*Practical Tip*

Wait 30 minutes after any change in ventilator settings before you check an arterial blood gas.

## Other parameters

Of course, there are lots of other things you may choose to monitor in any individual, such as level of consciousness. The ventilator may generate parameters you are interested in charting – leak, compliance, etc. Polysomnography is sometimes performed if it is particularly important to check if the patient is sleeping, for example when setting up NIV for long-term use at home.

## The ventilator display

Some ventilators just have the control buttons and knobs on the front, but many have some sort of indicator to show how the ventilator is working. One simple version is a dial with a pointer which shows the pressure within the ventilator. This will swing between inspiration and expiration, in the way we have seen in the pressure time traces earlier in this book. Another simple device is a bar which lights up to the height corresponding to pressure. With advances in computer technology, many modern ventilators have a graphical display. This might take the form of our pressure-time graph, often with flow at the same time. Add in a few icons to show you the mode of ventilation, some text with the backup settings and current estimated Vt or minute ventilation and we have what - at first glance - is a pretty intimidating display. Don't panic. It is possible to use the display to help you straight away, even if it will take some time before you are fully conversant with every aspect. Look at the main trace of pressure and time; when you are happy, look at flow; then see how the flow is used to calculate volume, if this is included on the display. Start at one side of the display and look at each item in turn, making a note of those you don't understand. If you don't think you need to know about them at this stage, then leave them and visit them another time; if you think they might be important for you to know about at this stage, then ask someone or look in the manual.

## Summary

- Look at the patient and the monitors.

- Monitoring of respiratory rate, pulse, blood pressure and $SpO_2$ will suffice for most patients starting NIV in the acute setting depending on the gender.

# 15
# Alarms

---

## Learning points

By the end of this chapter you should be able to

- Decide what alarms you want to use
- Set low pressure and high flow alarms
- *Explain how low pressure and high flow alarms detect disconnection*
- *Explain how low flow alarms detect occlusion*

---

If you ask patients who have been on ICU, they think that every time an alarm goes off they are going to die. They cannot tell if it is their alarm or another patient's. Unlike the ICU staff, they cannot distinguish between a ventilator disconnection alarm and an infusion pump that has finished. This happens to a lesser extent with NIV, but it is still important to think about what you want an alarm to tell you about. Alarms often start to go off whilst you are setting a patient up on NIV. This is annoying, distracting and also undermines the patient's confidence in you. Use the option on the ventilator to silence the alarms until you have the patient settled on NIV.

> **Key points**
>
> If an alarm is not going to be acted upon, it should be disabled.

## Ventilator malfunction

If there is an internal problem with the ventilator, an alarm will usually go off. The ventilator will probably have stopped working, so the patient may well have taken off their mask already and alerted you to the problem. An alarm will sound if the ventilator becomes unplugged, or if the power fails. If the ventilator has an internal battery, a light may come and/or there may be an intermittent audible alarm to tell you that at some stage in the next few hours you need to get the power supply sorted out. Power alarms are often the only sensible alarms on a ventilator, in that they alert you to an important problem that you might  not otherwise notice (ie that the ventilator has switched to its battery), they are usually acted on and are minimally intrusive to the clinical environment (often visible rather than audible).

## Low pressure

Low pressure alarms have traditionally been the method used to detect a problem with the ventilator circuit.  If you disconnect the circuit from a patient on NIV, the pressure-time trace will look like this:

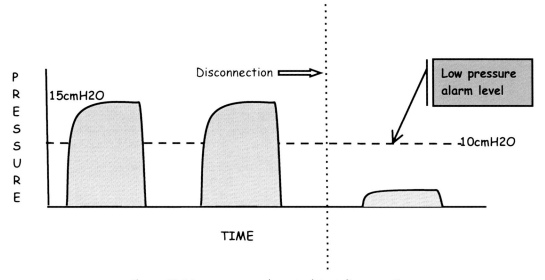

Figure 15.1 Low-pressure alarm to detect disconnection.

An alarm set to go off if the pressure during inspiration doesn't get to $10cmH_2O$ will detect this event.  Notice how the pressure is not zero, because there is some resistance to flow in the circuit – if the alarm had been set to zero, it would not go off.   For ventilator-dependent patients, it may be advisable to have an independent low pressure alarm that is not integral to the ventilator, just in case the ventilator packs up and the internal alarms also stop working.  These devices are more commonly used for patients ventilated through a tracheostomy.  You could use an oxygen saturation monitor, but this means that you will only be alerted some time after ventilation has stopped and you will have even less time to sort things out.

> ### *Practical Tip*
>
> If you are using low pressure to detect ventilator disconnection, check that the alarm goes off when you remove the mask from the patient.

## High flow

If we add flow to this example, you can see how the flow delivered by the ventilator shoots up when the disconnection occurs, as the ventilator tries to get the pressure up to the target IPAP:

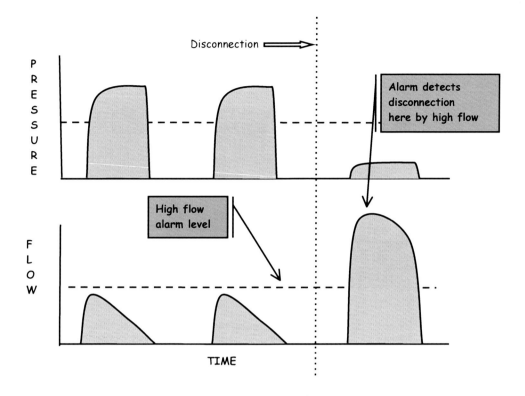

**Figure 15.2** High-flow alarm to detect disconnection.

Many BIPAP ventilators use high flow alarms to detect disconnection. Measuring flow also allows you to notice when a mask leak develops, because there is an increase in flow, even if there isn't much change in the pressure.

## Low flow

If the ventilator circuit is occluded, for example if secretions have clogged up a filter, then the target pressure will be reached with very little flow from the ventilator. Low flow alarms can also alert you to occlusion of the upper airway, again because the target pressure is reached too easily:

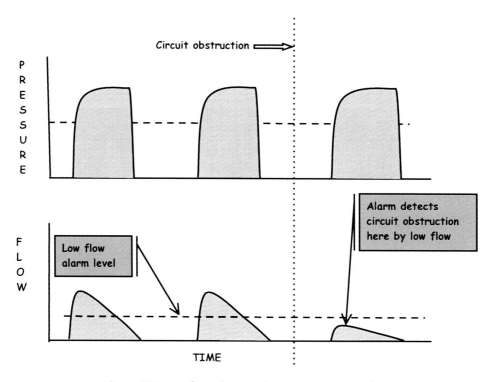

**Figure 15.3** Low-flow alarm to detect circuit obstruction.

## High pressure

During ventilation through an endotracheal tube, a high pressure alarm is needed to alert if excessively high pressures are being applied to the lung. With NIV, high pressures just blow the mask off the face, so a high pressure alarm is redundant. In a pressure-controlled or pressure support ventilator, there should not be a need for high pressure alarms, because the ventilator will not deliver pressures higher than the set pressure. In volume-controlled ventilation, a set volume is delivered; if the patient's condition deteriorates or the circuit becomes occluded, an alarm may be used to alert you to the excessively high pressures which are needed to maintain tidal volume.

## Tidal volume and minute ventilation

Volume controlled ventilators can give you a pretty accurate estimate of the volume of air delivered to the patient, and will alarm if this drops below any given level you specify. Some modern BIPAP ventilators also estimate volume.

## Alarms and mouthpiece NIV

When a patient is awake and using a mouthpiece for top-up assisted breaths during the day, for example whilst eating or holding a conversation, they do not need an alarm to tell them that they have taken the mouthpiece out of their mouth. An alarm constantly going off is going to be an irritation. Some patients just keep their cheek up against the mouthpiece when they are breathing through it, to keep the pressure above the alarm level. The mouthpiece causes a bit of resistance to flow, so there will usually be pressure within the circuit even when the patient is not connected. You can set the alarm below this level, but clearly it is important to increase the threshold again to detect disconnection during the night.

## Remote alarms

An alarm needs to alert someone to do something about the condition which has set the alarm off. This might be a carer elsewhere in the house for a patient using NIV at home, so the alarm needs to be very loud. Some ventilators will allow you to connect a remote loudspeaker using a long cable. Environmental control engineers will be able to help connect the ventilator to a remote alarm.

## Summary

- Alarms have a tendency to be more of a hindrance than a help.

- Keep it simple – use as few alarms as you can.

- A high flow alarm is probably the most useful – use it to tell you if the mask has become disconnected or dislodged.

# 16
# Triggering

**Learning points**

By the end of this chapter you should be able to:

* Describe how a patient can trigger a breath in.

* *Describe how a BIPAP ventilator decides when to switch from inspiration to expiration.*

* *Adjust trigger sensitivity.*

* *Define auto-triggering.*

**Keywords:**

Autotriggering

Most of the time, you won't need to touch the triggers on an NIV ventilator. When you are using NIPPV you don't really want the patient to be triggering many breaths themselves - the whole idea is for the ventilator to do most of the work. With BIPAP for acute respiratory failure, most patients will be fine with standard trigger settings.

## Mask leaks and triggering

Mask leaks have a bad effect on triggering. If the patient starts to take a breath in, most of the air comes from around the mask and is not sensed by the ventilator, which therefore fails to trigger inspiration. If the flow rate during inspiration is very high because of leaks, the reduction in the flow into the patient as their lungs fill up is only a small proportion of the excessively high flow: if the ventilator is looking for a proportional fall in flow, say to 30% of maximum, before triggering expiration, this will not happen and inspiration will probably be terminated when a maximum time has expired.

*Practical Tip*

Before you start adjusting trigger sensitivity, make sure that the mask fit is as good as you can get it.

## Triggering inspiration

All NIV ventilators will allow the patient to trigger the start of the next breath. In older ventilators this involves pressure triggering, where the patient has to generate a small negative pressure to tell the ventilator that they want to take a breath in. Most modern ventilators use flow triggers: when the ventilator detects a small inspiratory flow, this then activates inspiratory pressure generation. If you have a patient who is struggling to co-ordinate their breathing with the ventilator, you can try a more sensitive inspiratory trigger. Watch the patient breathing on the ventilator to make sure you haven't made the trigger so sensitive that it is triggering even when the patient isn't trying to breathe in (auto-triggering).

## Triggering expiration

In NIPPV, expiration is not triggered but occurs after a set amount of time. You choose this time, not the patient. Having watched the patient breathing spontaneously, you might choose an inspiratory time of 1.5 seconds and set the ventilator accordingly.

In BIPAP we have seen how the patient triggers the ventilator across from inspiration to expiration. Again this is best done by detecting a fall in flow rate – at the end of a breath in, there is less and less air entering the lungs, and when flow falls below a set level then it is time to withdraw the IPAP and change to expiration. Once again, you don't usually need to adjust the expiratory trigger.

In patients with COPD the peak expiratory flow may be very low, and it may take too long to reach 30% of this level. Increasing the cut-off to 50%, or even 70%, of maximum flow will be more comfortable for the patient - the flow levels may not be specified, but just marked as "sensitivity". Shortening inspiration will allow them more time to breathe out and reduce the chances of them becoming over-inflated. Watch carefully to check that they get a reasonable breath in, and don't switch across to expiration too early.

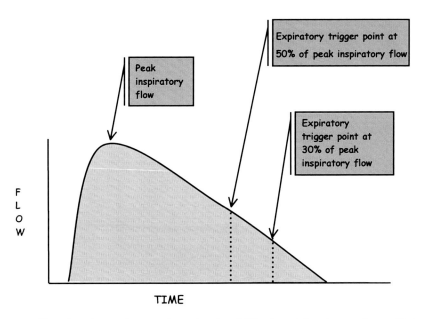

**Figure 16.1** Changing the expiratory trigger level to 50% of peak inspiratory flow will shorten the duration of inspiration.

There is always a maximum time set for inspiration, irrespective of what is happening to flow. This is a safety mechanism, so that the ventilator doesn't blow for thirty seconds whilst waiting for flow to reach a particular trigger level.

*How to do it*

**Adjust triggers**

- Check the mask and minimize leaks first before you adjust the triggers.
- Watch the patient on NIV.
- If they are having to make quite an effort to trigger a breath in, make the inspiratory trigger more sensitive.
- Watch again, and check that the setting is not so sensitive that the ventilator is sensing a breath when there isn't one (auto-triggering).
- The expiratory trigger needs to be more sensitive if the patient is having to contract their expiratory muscles to turn off inspiration, or if there is a long pause after the lungs are fully inflated before switching to expiration.
- Increase the flow level at which the switch to expiration occurs.
- Watch again, and check that inspiration is not now too short.

## Summary

- Most modern ventilators use flow to trigger the start of inspiration.
- During BIPAP expiration is triggered when inspiratory flow falls below a certain level.
- Mask leaks interfere with these triggers.

# 17

# Obesity-Hypoventilation

## Learning points

By the end of this chapter you should be able to

- Identify patients with central hypoventilation from their blood gases and spirometry.
- Select patients with obesity-hypoventilation for long-term NIV.
- Be able to set up NIV for these patients.
- *Explain about respiratory drive.*

## Keywords:

Central hypoventilation, Obesity-hypoventilation syndrome.

Many of the patients with COPD who do well on NIV are pretty overweight. They are "blue bloaters" rather than "pink puffers". Actually, they sometimes turn out to have COPD that isn't all that bad, and the cause of hypoventilation was more one of central respiratory drive. Many obese patients have poor respiratory drive – when they become hypercapnic this is termed the obesity-hypoventilation syndrome.

## Which patients?

Patients with muscle weakness, chest wall deformity or central respiratory drive problems sometimes present with acute or acute-on-chronic type 2 respiratory failure. In these patients, it doesn't matter what the pH level is: they need NIV. If you see an elevated $PaCO_2$ in a patient with any of these problems, then much the safest policy is to start NIV straight away. Don't be fooled by how well they look – if you do nothing then you are highly likely to get a call from ICU a few days later. I think you should apply the same principle to patients with obesity, with the proviso that some severe obstructive sleep apnoea patients (almost invariably with severe obesity) will be hypercapnic at presentation, but their $PaCO_2$ falls within a few weeks of starting CPAP; using NIV in these patients will not do them any harm, but might be overkill – you can always wean them to CPAP at a later date.

**Key point**

Obese patients with an elevated $PaCO_2$ are likely to need NIV at night in the long term

## What ventilator settings?

Start with BIPAP, but be prepared to switch to NIPPV if the patient doesn't pick up quickly. Respiratory drive is poor in these patients, particularly at night, so they will be using the back-up settings most of the time. This should be fine, but BIPAP ventilators are designed to support rather than provide ventilation, and they don't do the latter as well. If the patient takes very short shallow breaths at a rate above the back-up rate, the ventilator supports these breaths, but it may not provide adequate alveolar ventilation. If you do use BIPAP, start with an IPAP of 15cmH$_2$O or so, but push it up fairly soon to 20cmH$_2$O once the patient is settled. If they will tolerate it, you can use even higher IPAP, up to about 30cmH$_2$O. An EPAP of 5cmH$_2$O is fine to start with, but if the patient is very obese and oxygenation or upper airway obstruction is a problem, then you can increase this to 10cmH$_2$O. Set a reasonably high back-up rate (12 to 15/min) with an I:E ratio of 1:2 (unless the patient also has COPD, when 1:3 would be better).

If you use NIPPV, start with an IPAP of 20cmH$_2$O. The idea is to <u>provide</u> ventilation, not <u>support</u> the patient's own breathing. You want the patient to relax and let the ventilator do all the work, which they will find difficult to do if you start with an IPAP that is too low. Watch carefully to see if the patient is triggering the ventilator – try and get them not to trigger, by getting them to relax and by adjusting the ventilator settings. You may need to push the IPAP up to 30cmH$_2$O to get enough air in. Set the respiratory rate at (or just below) the patient's own spontaneous rate. If they are breathing very fast, which is unlikely in this setting, see if you can bring the rate down over the next few hours, aiming for 10-15 breaths per minute. Set the I:E ratio to that of the patient's own breathing pattern. You may be able to prolong inspiration a bit once they are settled on NIV, which will improve ventilation, but watch the patient carefully to make sure they still have time to breathe right out before the next breath comes along.

## Where?

These patients have often experienced a slow decline into respiratory failure, and tolerate terrible arterial blood gases surprisingly well. They are often fine on a respiratory ward, but the very sick ones should be on HDU.

## How long for?

Very occasionally, a patient with obesity-hypoventilation will lose a massive amount of weight and be able to stop using NIV. Most patients will need to continue with nocturnal NIV indefinitely.

## Alveolar ventilation and PaCO₂

The amount of $CO_2$ washed out of the lungs is dependant on the alveolar ventilation – the amount of air getting to the gas-exchanging parts of the lungs. If alveolar ventilation is reduced, then less $CO_2$ is washed out and $PaCO_2$ rises. The relationship between alveolar ventilation and $PaCO_2$ is not linear: at low levels of alveolar ventilation, any further reduction will result in a much larger rise in $PaCO_2$.

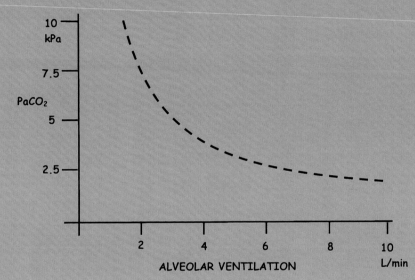

**Figure 17.1** A similar change in alveolar ventilation will result in a much larger change in $PaCO_2$ if alveolar ventilation is already low.

## Other central hypoventilation syndromes

Central hypoventilation is a common reason for starting NIV in children. NIPPV is usually the best mode. If the main problem is central drive, without any associated obesity or chest wall deformity, then an IPAP of 15cmH₂O will be sufficient. Overnight monitoring of $CO_2$ is important to check that ventilation is adequate, but also to ensure that you don't hyperventilate the patient.

## Respiratory drive

You can measure respiratory drive by filling a large bag (20 litres or so) with oxygen and breathing in and out of it for a few minutes. There will be sufficient oxygen to prevent your $SpO_2$ dropping, but $CO_2$ will build up in the bag. As you start to rebreathe this $CO_2$, your $PaCO_2$ will rise. This will stimulate your respiratory centre and make you breathe deeper and faster. You can measure the slope of the increase in ventilation as $CO_2$ rises. If your respiratory drive is poor, you will see a much smaller increase in ventilation:

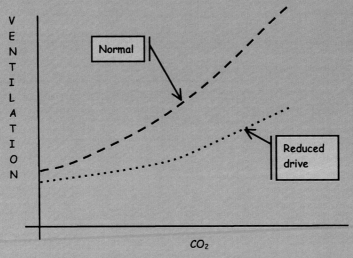

**Figure 17.2** Ventilatory response to increasing carbon dioxide.

Normally, hypercapnia is a more important factor than hypoxia in driving respiration. In chronic type 2 respiratory failure, the respiratory centre gets used to a high $CO_2$ (and any increase in $CO_2$ is buffered by the large "pool" of bicarbonate) – hypoxic drive becomes more important. Abolishing hypoxic drive – by administering supplementary oxygen – will reduce ventilation even further.

The increase in ventilation depends not only on respiratory drive, but also on how easy it is to get air in and out of the lungs. One way of overcoming this difficulty is to block off the mouthpiece – without the patient knowing – and measure the pressure 0.1 seconds after they start trying to take a breath in. This is called P0.1. There is no flow if the mouthpiece is blocked off, so the mechanics of how difficult it is to get air into the lungs is irrelevant. In practice, measuring respiratory drive is quite difficult. As with lung compliance, the normal ranges are not well defined.

## Summary

- Start NIV in any patient with severe obesity who is hypercapnic, unless there is a good reason not to.
- Ignore the pH level.
- Start with BIPAP, but change to NIPPV if the patient doesn't improve rapidly.
- Start with a pressure of 20cmH$_2$O.
- Continue with NIV at night in the long term.

# 18

# Respiratory rate

## BIPAP

Most of the time, a patient on BIPAP will dictate their own respiratory rate. If they were to stop breathing (for example a patient with chronic respiratory failure who is given too much oxygen) then we want the ventilator to kick in with a back-up rate. Common settings are about 10-12 breaths per minute. Twelve breaths per minute means one breath every five seconds. In the next figure, the patient stops breathing after the third breath; when five seconds have elapsed since the start of the previous breath, the back-up rate of the ventilator kicks in. Sometimes these breaths initiated by the ventilator are called mandatory or control breaths.

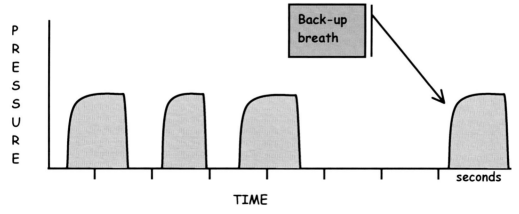

**Figure 18.1** In BIPAP, respiratory rate refers to the back-up rate at which the ventilator will deliver a breath if the patient stops breathing.

If the patient does not improve on your initial settings, one possible way of improving ventilation is to increase the back-up rate until the ventilator is going faster than the patient's spontaneous rate. In practice, playing around with the back-up settings on a BIPAP ventilator seldom seems to do much for gas exchange, perhaps because that is not what the ventilator was primarily designed to do. If you want to dictate what sort of breath is delivered, use NIPPV.

### Key points

During BIPAP, the respiratory rate setting is the back-up rate, below which the ventilator will start to deliver breaths without being triggered.

### Physiology

### Respiratory Rate

Faster rated with smaller volumes mean less elastic work or breathing, as less energy is expended stretching the lung and ribcage, like an elastic band, with each breath

Slower rates mean less "resistance" work pushing air in and out of the airways, because there is more time for air to get into the lungs and so flow rates are lower.

The total work of breathing is the sum of elastic and resistance work. Patients automatically choose the best rate for their particular combination of compliance and resistance, to minimize the amount of energy they use in breathing:

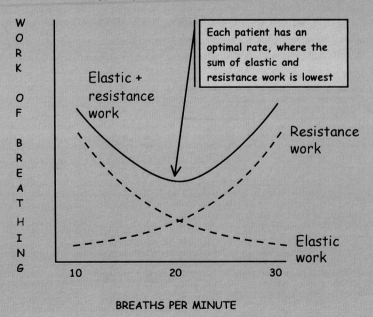

Fig 18.2 Total work of breathing at different respiratory rates.

If a patient's lungs are very stiff (ie compliance is low), then the work of breathing is lower when they breathe with rapid shallow breaths. There are two problems with fast respiratory rates:

- A greater proportion of the small volume breaths is wasted on dead space
- More ventilation goes to "fast" alveoli with short time constants. We'll look at this point in the next chapter.

## NIPPV

With NIPPV, the ventilator determines the timing of each breath as well as the target pressure. Set the rate at, or just below, the patient's own rate. This will often be quite fast, but if you try and start with a slower rate the patient will probably struggle to co-ordinate with the ventilator. The rate can be slowed down as the patient's clinical condition improves.

## Summary

- During BIPAP you don't need to worry too much about respiratory rate, but set a reasonable back-up rate
- When starting NIPPV, set the respiratory rate at the patient's own spontaneous rate. Slow the rate down gradually.

# 19

# Inspiratory:expiratory ratio

## Learning points

By the end of this chapter you should be able to:

- Set the I:E ratio for back-up breaths in BIPAP according to the presence or absence of airflow obstruction.
- *Set the I:E ratio for NIPPV.*
- *Explain how short expiratory times lead to hyperinflation.*
- *Calculate the I:E ratio from respiratory rate and inspiratory time.*

During tidal breathing, you spend about a third of the time breathing in, then a third breathing out; the final third is a pause before the next breath in. If one third of the breathing cycle is spent breathing in and two thirds breathing out (including the pause as part of expiration), this gives an I:E ratio of 1:2.

When a patient develops breathing problems, they pinch time from the pause between breaths and start the next breath as soon as the previous breath finishes. If they have a problem with getting air out of the lungs, for example COPD, the pause will be used for expiration. If the problem is getting air into the lungs, for example in neuromuscular weakness, more time will be spent in inspiration.

During spontaneous breathing, patients automatically breathe with the I:E ratio which is most efficient for them. With BIPAP, the ventilator will allow them to breathe with this pattern too, except for back-up breaths. Use a ratio of 1:2 for the back-up breaths, or 1:3 if the patient has airflow obstruction.

### Key point

In BIPAP, the I:E ratio setting only applies to back-up breaths.

## NIPPV

### Inspiratory time

Start with the same time as the patient takes for a spontaneous breath. Watch the patient carefully on NIPPV (and/or look at the volume-time trace on the ventilator if there is one) and adjust the inspiratory time so that it is just long enough for the lungs to reach full inflation. If you try and prolong inspiration too much, then the patient will start to feel uncomfortable and start to fight the ventilator. Once the patient is settled, you will probably be able to slow the rate down. One way of doing this is just to increase the inspiratory time a little. If you watch the patient, you will probably be able to see that the chest expands better. There comes a point, however, where the chest has expanded as much as it is going to for that IPAP – prolonging inspiration further will be uncomfortable for the patient, even though it might allow time for air to get into the bits of lung with long time constants.

*Physiology*

**Alveolar time constants**

Stiff areas of lung - with reduced compliance – have short time constants and are sometimes called "fast" alveolar units. They inflate very quickly. A high elastic recoil pressure (which is the same thing as reduced compliance) stops airways collapsing, so this part of the lung will also empty very quickly.

With a rapid respiratory rate, more ventilation will go to these "fast" parts of the lung. They may not be very good at getting oxygen across into the blood as the "slower" areas of normal lung.

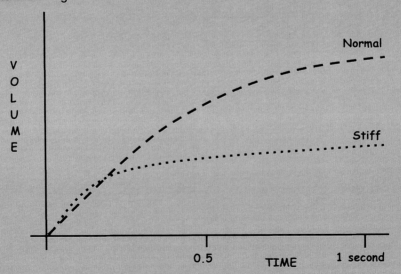

**Figure 19.1** The time taken to inflate alveoli with low compliance is shorter than for normal areas of lung.

Just to complete the picture, in COPD there will be very slow alveolar units, with long time constants. This is because they have narrow airways and very compliant (emphysematous) alveoli.

## Expiratory time

Someone with fairly normal lungs will have completed expiration in about a second or two. In severe COPD, expiration may take three seconds or more. It is essential that you leave enough time for these patients to exhale, but again this should be apparent by watching the patient carefully. If you have the luxury of a flow trace, you can see whether or not expiratory flow falls to zero before the next breath in:

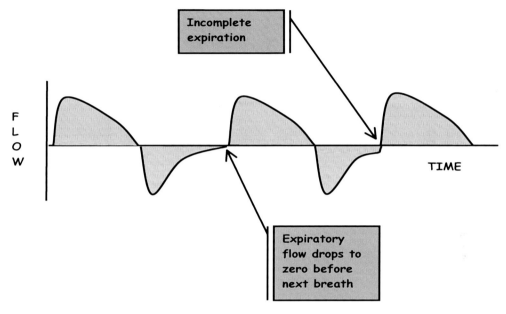

**Fig 19.2** Expiratory flow. Inspecting the expiratory flow on the flow-time trace will show you if there is sufficient time for expiration to complete before the next breath. This applies for "control" breaths – during BIPAP the patient will determine the optimal expiratory time for themselves.

If you don't allow the patient to complete expiration, you will progressively hyperinflate them. PEEPi will become more of a problem (see "Triggering"). Try breathing for a minute or so just below total lung capacity rather than your normal lung volume - it is uncomfortable, and harder work for your inspiratory muscles.

*Terminology*

**I:E ratio**

Some ventilators give you the respiratory rate, then allow you to adjust the I:E ratio. For example, if you choose a rate of 15 breaths per minute, each breath will be four seconds long; an I:E ratio of 1:3 means inspiration would last one second and expiration three seconds. Other ventilators get you to set the inspiratory and expiratory times separately. So we might set inspiration to 1.5 seconds and expiration to 3 seconds; total breath time is 4.5 seconds, the I:E ratio is 1:2 and the rate is just over 13 breaths per minute (60/4.5).

## Summary

- I:E ratio means the ratio of the time spent in inspiration to that spent in expiration
- Don't worry too much about I:E ratios on BIPAP – they only apply to the back-up rate
- In NIPPV, set the I:E ratio to the pattern of spontaneous breathing
- In  COPD you will need a long expiratory time, and you may need to shorten the inspiratory time to get an appropriate I:E ratio

# 20

# Type 1 Respiratory Failure

**Learning points:**

By the end of this chapter you should be able to:

*   Identify patients with type 1 respiratory failure who might benefit from NIV.

*   Ensure that NIV for these patients is delivered in an appropriate clinical area.

*   *Describe how you would bronchoscope a patient on NIV.*

NIV helps with ventilation rather than oxygenation, but some patients with type 1 respiratory failure (low $PaO_2$, normal or low $PaCO_2$) seem to benefit. The evidence suggests that it is better to start it early, and then intubate if NIV fails. NIV doesn't work at all well when it is used as a last-ditch option, when the patient has been turned down for intubation by ICU, on a "nothing to lose" basis.

> ***Key point***
>
> If you are going to use NIV in type 1 respiratory failure, start it early

## Which patients?

The list of conditions for which NIV has been documented to be effective is getting longer and includes pneumonia, trauma, adult respiratory distress syndrome (ARDS), severe acute respiratory syndrome (SARS) and asthma. The level of evidence for the use of NIV in these conditions is not yet particularly high, although there is an accumulating body of evidence in immunocompromised patients with diffuse lung infiltrates.

**Bronchoscope during NIV**

You may need to bronchoscope a patient whilst they are on NIV, either to lavage in order to get a diagnosis in a patient with diffuse infiltrates, or to remove a plug of sputum which is causing a segment of lung to collapse.

- Obtain consent.
- Keep the patient nil-by-mouth for four hours before the procedure.
- Decide if it going to be safe to use sedation.
- Make sure you have good intravenous access.
- Check all the endoscopic equipment carefully before you start.
- Make sure everything you might possibly need is at hand.
- Turn the supplementary oxygen up to maximum.
- Insert a bronchoscopy connector (available from ICU) where the circuit attaches to the mask. If you have one available, use a special NIV bronchoscopy mask or helmet.
- Double-check that everything is ready.
- Insert the bronchoscope.
- Be as quick as you can. If you have prepared carefully, you can do a bronchoalveolar lavage in a minute or so. Getting plugs of sputum out of a collapsed lobe may take longer.

## What settings?

Use BIPAP. Since the patient has difficulty with oxygenation, you will need to use a high EPAP such as 10cmH$_2$O. The lungs are stiff, so IPAP needs to be a lot higher than this to increase ventilation, say 25cmH$_2$O. Add supplementary oxygen to keep the SpO$_2$ above 90%.

## Where?

There is a high likelihood of needing to intubate, so patients with type 1 respiratory failure should receive NIV on ICU. If intubation is not an option, it may be appropriate to use HDU. These patients may become severely hypoxic if their mask comes off, so they should not be managed on a lower intensity facility such as general or respiratory ward.

## How long for?

As with COPD, it should be apparent within a few hours if NIV is going to work. If gas exchange has not improved after four hours, you should probably stop and consider intubation.

## Alveolar-arterial oxygen difference

To see how good the lungs are at getting oxygen across into the blood, calculate the alveolar oxygen level and compare it with that in the arterial blood: if there is a big discrepancy, then the lungs are not working well. The bigger the discrepancy, the less likely NIV is to work. To calculate this you use the alveolar gas equation again:

$$PAO_2 = (FiO_2 \times 94) - (1.25 \times PaCO_2)$$

The alveolar-arterial difference ($PAO_2 - PaO_2$) is normally about 1kPa. It becomes much larger when the lungs are diseased. The most important cause is ventilation/perfusion imbalance. The reason for this is simple to understand if you look at two alveolar units in Figure 20.1, one of which is very poorly perfused (Unit A) and the other of which is poorly ventilated (Unit B). Since there is very little perfusion of Unit A, the composition of gas within it will be quite similar to inspired air – the $PAO_2$ will be high, and the blood leaving the unit will be well-oxygenated. On the other hand Unit B is under-ventilated, so the blood leaving the unit is little different from the blood entering it – poorly-oxygenated mixed venous blood. So, we have well -oxygenated blood leaving Unit A and poorly-oxygenated blood leaving Unit B. The two sources of blood mix together in pulmonary veins, ready to be transported round the arterial system. We already noted that Unit A was under-perfused, so most of the blood comes from Unit B which is poorly oxygenated.

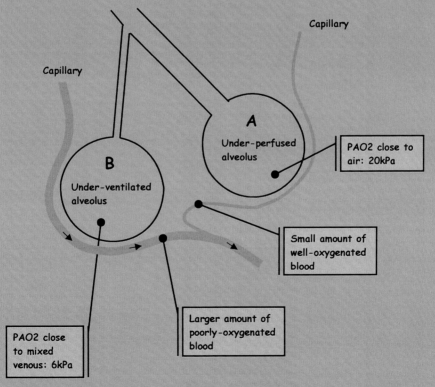

**Figure 20.1** Ventilation/Perfusion imbalance. A larger proportion of the blood entering the systemic arterial system comes from Unit B which is under-ventilated but well-perfused, in comparison with Unit A which is well-ventilated but under-perfused.

## Summary

- NIV can work in carefully selected patients with type 1 respiratory failure
- Start it early
- Don't delay intubation if NIV doesn't work

# 21

# Complications

---

**Learning points**

By the end of this chapter you should be able to:

- List potential complications of NIV.

- Add a humidifier to a NIV circuit.

- *Plan how you would assess and reduce the risk of complications in your unit.*

---

Serious complications of NIV are pretty rare. Skin problems and nasal symptoms are more common, and often limit how much NIV your patient will tolerate.

## Nasal bridge pressure sores

The most common complication is skin ulceration because of pressure from the mask. The bridge of the nose has very little tissue between the cartilage and the skin, and can easily become red or ulcerated within a few hours on NIV particularly if the mask straps are very tight. Prevention is better than cure. Don't over-tighten masks. If the skin starts to become red then change to a different style of mask before ulceration develops – this might be a smaller mask which fits over the tip of the nose, one with a pad which sits on the forehead to relieve pressure on the nasal bridge, or some nasal pillows. Some units routinely apply a small square of protective dressing such as Granuflex to the bridge of the nose in a patient starting NIV acutely who is likely to have a mask on for most of the first 24 hours.

## Nasal symptoms

Sneezing is sometimes a problem when a patient first starts NIV, probably because the higher flow rates during ventilation cool down the nose. Some patients on long term NIV continue to experience lots of nasal symptoms, such as stuffiness or a runny nose. Steroid or anticholinergic nasal sprays may be helpful. They should be tried for several weeks, applied to each nostril twice daily. Other simple measures include an insulating sleeve around the ventilator tubing, or putting a few drops of decongestant in the bacterial filter each night. If none of these measures work, increasing the humidity of the inspired air may be worth a try.

Sometimes a device called a heat and moisture exchanger (HME) is used in ICU to humidify the inspired air. This works by using a filter to condense the water out of the exhaled air (in the same way as water condenses out of your breath when you breathe out against a cold glass window); when the dry gas from the ventilator passes through this filter on its way to the patient, it picks up water and increases its humidity. HMEs will easily block if the patient has any secretions, and may also become saturated with water. The resistance of the HME may then be very high, which isn't a problem for the ventilator to overcome, but may make it very difficult for the patient to generate enough flow to trigger the ventilator. The best way to increase humidity during NIV is to use a heated humidifier.

**How to do it**

**Humidify with NIV**

- Use a length of 22mm tubing to connect the ventilator outlet to the humidifier inlet.
- Connect the NIV circuit to the humidifier outlet
- In NIPPV, you will need to detach the exhalation valve and patient trigger tubing from the larger tubing, so they can run directly to the ventilator.

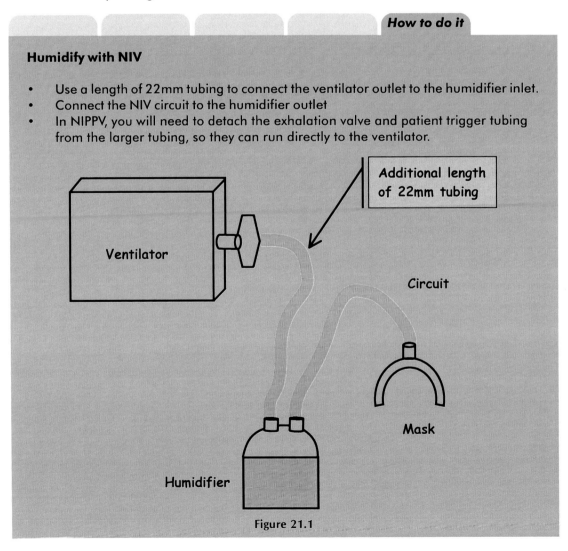

Figure 21.1

## Sinus pain

Some patients experience pain in their sinuses during NIV. Apart from reducing the IPAP, it is difficult to do much about this.

## Irritation of eyes

If a mask fits badly, sometimes the air blowing into the eyes can cause irritation. Try a better-fitting mask.

## Gastric distension

When you apply pressure to the upper airway through a mask, most of the air will go into the lungs but some may go down into the oesophagus. Patients on long-term NIV learn to stop this from happening, although quite how they do so is not clear.

## Oesophageal perforation

There have been occasional reports of oesophageal rupture on NIV, in patients who had a spontaneous perforation some years previously. NIV should not be used soon after oesophageal or gastric surgery.

## Pneumothorax

Pneumothorax as a complication of NIV is extremely rare, but something to bear in mind if a patient deteriorates suddenly. It is more likely to occur in someone with bullous or cystic lung disease. It is possible to continue with NIV in the presence of a small pneumothorax, but it is much safer to insert a chest drain.

## Facial shape

Use of a mask for hours at a time will distort the shape of the face, particularly in children. Nasal pillows may cause dilation of the anterior nares. Prolonged use of a mouthpiece can alter the alignment of teeth.

## Summary

- Serious complications of NIV are rare.
- Nasal bridge pressure is the most common problem.

# 22

# Failure of NIV

**Learning points**

By the end of this chapter you should be able to:

- Decide what to do when your patient is not improving on NIV.

- *Explain when and how you would use sedation with NIV.*

After an hour or so, a patient you have started on NIV should begin to improve. Often this is apparent from the end of the bed, in that they no longer look as if they are fighting to stay alive. An arterial blood gas sample will tell you if your clinical impression is right. If the pH level and $PaCO_2$ are moving in the right direction, then you need do nothing more – changing the ventilator settings or mask may well unsettle the patient, just when they are getting used to NIV.

Sometimes the patient seems to be better when you look at them and their gases are also improving, but when you watch them being ventilated it is clear that NIV is not working. They may be out of synchronisation with the ventilator, or there are lots of leaks and the target pressure isn't being achieved, or they are just unhappy about the whole thing and trying to pull the mask off the whole time. In this case they are improving <u>despite</u> rather than because of NIV, and you should discontinue it.

> **Key points**
>
> There is always a danger of persevering with NIV too long. Don't delay intubation if it is apparent that NIV is not going to work.

What if the patient does not look any better and their arterial blood gases are not improving? It may be best to abandon NIV, but there are a few things to check first.

## Is the patient breathing in time with the ventilator?

If the patient is not synchronising with the ventilator, then NIV will not be achieving anything, and may even be making the situation worse. The most common problem is mask leak, but there are a few other things you could try:

- Check the circuit is connected correctly. If you are using NIPPV, check that the smaller tubes are connected at both ends, and not blocked by water or secretions.

- Check that the filter has not become clogged with water or secretions.

- Increase the inspiratory trigger sensitivity.

- Increase EPAP if the patient has COPD, to overcome PEEPi.

- If the patient is breathing very fast, shorten the rise time.

- Increase the EPAP, if you think that upper airway obstruction is occurring. This is more likely to occur when the patient is asleep. See what happens if you change the position of the patient's head, if you pull their jaw forward or if you wake them up. You may need to sit them more upright. A nasopharyngeal airway may help if the patient's conscious level is impaired.

### Practical Tip

The commonest cause of patient-ventilator asynchrony is mask leak.

## Is the chest expansion adequate?

If the chest is expanding in time with the ventilator but the $PaCO_2$ is not improving:

- Think about re-breathing: check the patency of the expiratory port, use a different port.

- Increase the IPAP.

- Decrease the EPAP. This will increase span and hence Vt.

- With NIPPV, increase the inspiratory time.

- With NIPPV – or if the back-up rate is being used on BIPAP - increase the respiratory rate.

- Change ventilator mode. If you are not winning on BIPAP, try NIPPV. If these pressure-targeted modes aren't working, some patients will pick up on volume ventilation, but set a clear time limit on further trials of different modes.

### Practical Tip

In a patient with acute respiratory failure, think about fixed upper airway obstruction (eg by tumour or vocal cord abductor paralysis) if you cannot inflate the chest at all with NIV.

## Is medical therapy optimal?

Check that you have ordered all the appropriate medication, and that it has been given. It is easy to overlook things that you would routinely give if the patient wasn't on NIV. If it has been difficult to settle the patient onto NIV, there may not have been time to give them all their drugs. If the oxygen flow rate is too high, you may lose the patient's own contribution to ventilation. Aim for an $SpO_2$ of 88-92%.

## Have any complications developed?

Although very unlikely, it is always worth thinking about the possibility of a pneumothorax. If in doubt, get a chest X-ray. New lung shadowing might also indicate that the patient has aspirated.

## Would sedation help?

Very occasionally you may need to try sedating the patient to see if this improves their tolerance of NIV, but only do this if you are not going to proceed to intubation, or in an environment where the patient can be intubated rapidly if things deteriorate.

*How to do it*

**Sedate a patient on NIV**

- Use the intravenous route.
- Give small incremental doses every few minutes.
- Use a drug whose effect you can completely reverse, such as a benzodiazepine.
- Make sure the reversing agent is by the bedside.
- Remember that the half-life of the reversing agent is much shorter than the sedating drug - you may need to use repeat doses or even an infusion.

## Withdrawing NIV and palliative care

If the patient's clinical condition and their blood gases are deteriorating despite optimal NIV and a decision has been made not to intubate, then you should stop NIV. Do this as soon as it is clear that NIV is failing. The longer you delay this decision the more difficult it will be to stop NIV. The patient will usually be relieved to take off the mask. Sometimes they feel very breathless without NIV, but it is better to use oxygen, opiates or benzodiazepines to manage this rather than go back onto NIV. If the patient is dying, it is important that they are able to talk to their family and to the staff caring for them - NIV makes this difficult. It may also draw out the process of dying and prolong suffering.

It can be difficult to know how quickly a patient will deteriorate when you stop NIV, so make sure that all the right people are around.

If the patient cannot cope with stopping NIV so suddenly, try reducing the IPAP slowly. If you can get it down to less than $10cmH_2O$, the switch to spontaneous breathing may be less abrupt. This sounds kinder, but the whole process runs the risk of becoming very drawn out. NIV can prolong as well as alleviate suffering.

## Summary

- If a patient is not improving on NIV, watch them closely for a few minutes and diagnose the problem.

- If corrective action doesn't work, consider changing ventilator mode.

- The decision to intubate or palliate will depend on whether effective ventilation has been established with NIV.

# 23

# Neuromuscular Problems

**Learning points**

By the end of this chapter you should be able to:

*   List some examples of neuromuscular diseases which lead to chronic type 2 respiratory failure.

*   *Decide when a patient with one of these diseases needs NIV.*

*   *Discuss the circumstances where NIV can be used safely in acute neurological syndromes.*

We talked earlier on about splitting patients who need NIV into three groups:

1.  Patients with common diseases who present with acute hypercapnic respiratory failure and need NIV for a few hours or days during the acute illness (mainly COPD and LVF).

2.  Patients with fairly normal lungs who slip into hypercapnic respiratory failure because their breathing muscles give up or their central respiratory drive is poor (ventilatory pump failure).

3.  The rest.

Numerically, patients with ventilatory pump failure are much less common than our first group, but they are important to think about because a high proportion will need NIV subsequently at home. Long-term survival in these patients is often excellent, for example over 80% at five years in scoliosis or stable neuromuscular conditions, so it is important that you know how to get them through the initial crisis.

Type 2 respiratory failure – failure of ventilation – can occur because the load on the respiratory muscles is too great, or because the muscles are weak with a reduced capacity.

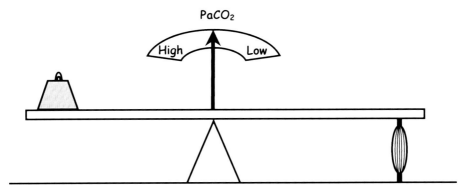

**Figure 23.1.** The balance between load and capacity determines whether a normal $PaCO_2$ can be maintained.

There are many diseases which can affect the respiratory muscles, either because the muscles themselves are involved, or because there is a problem with the nerves or neuromuscular junction. The end result is the same – respiratory muscles which don't contract. The clinical picture will depend upon which respiratory muscles are not working, and the degree of weakness.

---

### Practical Tip

If the vital capacity (VC) of a patient with a neuromuscular problem is greater than 1.5 L, the risk of them developing ventilatory failure is low

---

As a general rule, hypercapnic respiratory failure is unlikely unless inspiratory muscle strength is less than 50% predicted. This corresponds to a maximal inspiratory pressure (MIP) or sniff nasal inspiratory pressure (SNIP) of about $40cmH_2O$ (4kPa). Look and see if the patient is using their accessory muscles (sternomastoid etc) to breathe with at rest – a sign that all the main respiratory muscles are very weak - and count the respiratory rate: 30 breaths or more per minute implies that the muscles are so weak that Vt is small and the only way the patient can get a reasonable minute ventilation is by breathing very fast.

---

### How to do it

**Diagnose bilateral diaphragm paralysis**

- Ask the patient what happens to their breathing when they lie down. Normally, you increase the tone in your diaphragm when you lie down – if a patient is unable to do this, the contents of their abdomen push up into their ribcage and make them breathless.
- Ask them if they sleep propped up in bed. Patients with bilateral diaphragm paralysis sleep propped up on lots of pillows, or in a chair.
- Watch for paradoxical abdominal motion (inward motion during inspiration, because the diaphragm is passively sucked up into the thorax, as opposed to the normal pattern of active descent which pushes the anterior abdominal wall outwards) during quiet breathing.

- Put your hand on the patient's epigastric region, feel for paradox when you ask them to sniff.
- Lie the patient down and look again for paradox during tidal breathing; feel again for paradox when they sniff.
- Measure VC seated and lying. If the lying value is more than 15% lower, then this is a pointer to diaphragm paralysis.
- Measure MIP, SNIP and MEP. In isolated diaphragm paralysis, MIP and SNIP are low but MEP is normal. If MEP is also reduced, this indicates expiratory muscle involvement.
- If you are still in doubt, measure oesophageal and gastric pressures, using pressure transducers or balloons. Normally, diaphragmatic contraction leads to a positive gastric pressure during inspiration.

We try very hard to keep our $PaCO_2$ within the normal range, so if a patient with neuromuscular disease is hypercapnic during the daytime it means they have very weak respiratory muscles and will need NIV as a matter of urgency.

**Key points**

Hypercapnia is a very late development in neuromuscular patients. Start NIV the same day (or make plans for palliative care).

We all underventilate slightly when we are asleep; in neuromuscular disease, significant hypercapnia is often present first during sleep, and only manifests during the daytime as the disease progresses. Nocturnal awakenings and excessive daytime sleepiness may alert you to nocturnal hypoventilation in a patient, but the symptoms can be very vague – fatigue, poor appetite, weight loss, poor concentration, personality change.

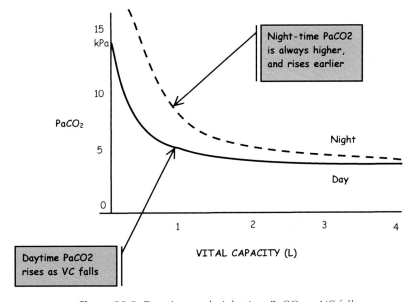

**Figure 23.2** Day-time and night-time $PaCO_2$ as VC falls

**Mouth pressures**

Maximum inspiratory and expiratory mouth pressures (MIP and MEP) are often used to estimate respiratory muscle strength. SNIP is also useful: the patient sniffs through one nostril whilst a pressure probe records the pressure in the other (occluded) nostril. For MIP, MEP and SNIP you can use:

- >80cmH$_2$O          Normal
- 40-80cmH$_2$O          Mild weakness
- 20-39cmH$_2$O          Moderate weakness
- <20cmH$_2$O          Severe weakness

## What mode and settings?

NIPPV is usually the best mode of NIV to use in neuromuscular patients. Even the effort of triggering the ventilator on and off is a considerable effort for these patients, and it is better to take over breathing for them completely. Set the respiratory rate slightly lower than their own rate, and think about adjusting this down as they improve. Patients with neuromuscular diseases are often very relieved to get onto NIV, and spontaneous respiratory effort will cease if you get their settings right. The chest will be fairly easy to inflate, so an IPAP of 15cmH$_2$O may be sufficient.

BIPAP is designed to support breathing rather than provide ventilation, and the back-up settings are only there as a safety measure. Neuromuscular patients will generate shallow, short breaths, particularly during sleep when the pattern may also be very irregular; the ventilator will support these breaths, but ventilation may well be inadequate because of the short inspiratory time unless spontaneous breathing stops altogether and the back-up settings kick in. EPAP makes triggering easy for COPD patients, but we aren't asking our neuromuscular patients to trigger the ventilator. EPAP will help keep the lungs inflated and overcome basal atelectasis, but pressure-controlled ventilation will also be adequate for this. For very weak patients, the effort of overcoming even a low EPAP can be quite a struggle.

**Practical Tip**

Patients with neuromuscular problems have pretty compliant chests, so be careful not to overventilate them.

# Which diseases?

## Muscle diseases

NIV works well in patients with muscle disorders such as muscular dystrophy. The classification of these disorders is evolving with the discovery of new genetic defects, but the current names of those which are particularly prone to affect the respiratory muscles are:

- Duchenne muscular dystrophy.
- Acid maltase deficiency.
- Limb-girdle muscular dystrophy.
- Nemaline myopathy.

You are likely to think about respiratory muscle weakness when the patient is already in a wheelchair because of limb muscle problems, but remember that some muscle diseases may have respiratory failure as their presenting problem. Some examples of muscle diseases where respiratory failure may occur when the patient is still ambulant are:

- Acid maltase deficiency.
- Emery-Dreifuss myopathy.
- Nemaline myopathy.
- Mitochondrial myopathy.
- Limb-girdle muscular dystrophy (type 2i).
- Minicore myopathy.

It isn't necessary (or possible, for most of us) to remember all the details of these different diseases, but you need to keep a closer eye on patients with a condition on any of the above two lists. An annual VC will be fine initially. When the VC falls below 1.5 litres, consider seeing them more often. An annual sleep study is also advisable at this stage. We used to wait until the patient had symptoms attributable to nocturnal hypoventilation before doing sleep studies, on the grounds that "prophylactic" NIV in patients without sleep disturbance was seldom tolerated. The problem is that these symptoms are sometimes very vague, and creep up on patients without them realising. Also, we now know that patients with neuromuscular diseases with asymptomatic nocturnal hypoventilation will be in trouble within a year or so. It is much better to start NIV before there is a crisis.

### Practical Tip

Remember to do regular echocardiograms on patients with muscle conditions that may affect the heart: Duchenne, Becker, Emery-Dreifuss, limb-girdle (type 1b) muscular dystrophies.

**The Tension Time Index**

Muscles get fatigued if they are asked to do too much work with insufficient time for recovery between each contraction. Imagine if you were asked to lift a really heavy weight once an hour; you might be able to manage it, but what would happen if you had to lift it every thirty seconds? For the respiratory muscles, we can calculate the tension time index. The first part of the equation is inspiratory time as a fraction of total breath time – if a high proportion of the total breath time is taken up by inspiration, there isn't much time for the muscles to recover before the next breath in. The second part of the equation is the load/capacity balance we have discussed before – the force generated during each breath in, as a proportion of the maximum strength of the inspiratory muscles:

Tension Time Index =
(Inspiratory time/total breath time) x (tidal inspiratory pressure/maximum inspiratory pressure)

The tidal inspiratory pressure is quite difficult to measure, unless you have a pressure probe in the oesophagus, but we could use the ratio of tidal volume to vital capacity.or

(Inspiratory time/total breath time) x (tidal volume/vital capacity)

It doesn't really matter what the critical value of the Tension Time Index is, but it is important to understand the concept that the timing of breathing and the proportion of maximum available force used are both key determinants of muscle fatigue.

**Motor neurone disease**

NIV is ideal for the minority of patients with motor neurone disease (MND) who develop respiratory failure with no or minimal bulbar involvement, particularly those who have disabling orthopnoea from diaphragm paralysis. This is usually associated with symptomatic sleep disturbance, and patients feel much better when they use NIV at night. As with muscle diseases, respiratory failure is unlikely if the VC is above 1.5 litres. Supine VC is better than sitting in this regard, but many patients find it difficult to get on and off a couch. Watch out for patients whose VC falls by more than 500mls between clinic visits – usually every 2-3 months in MND – and consider a trial of NIV before they get into trouble. NIV doesn't work well when the bulbar muscles are very weak. If bulbar problems are mild, it may be worth a trial of NIV: those in whom it is possible to establish effective ventilation will tend to live longer. Again as with muscular dystrophy, an elevated $PaCO_2$ implies critical respiratory muscle weakness: start NIV, or make a plan about intubation, resuscitation, palliative care, etc.

**Cervical cord lesions**

The diaphragm is innervated from cervical root segments C3, 4 and 5. Patients with a high cervical cord lesion will require a tracheostomy and full time ventilatory support. Those with slightly lower lesions may have some diaphragm function, which is enough to get them through the day, but they may need NIV at night.  Do an overnight sleep study and consider NIV if there are symptoms of sleep disturbance, if the daytime $PaCO_2$ is high, or if the patient has frequent respiratory tract infections  (which can be a sign of poor respiratory reserve in neuromuscular patients).

**Key point**

If patients with neuromuscular problems have more than three chest infections a year, this may be an indication that they need nocturnal NIV.

**Acute neurological syndromes**

There are some neurological diseases which cause acute paralysis which then improves either spontaneously or with treatment – polymyositis, ascending neuropathy (Guillain-Barre syndrome), myasthenia etc.  If ventilatory failure develops, intubation or tracheostomy are usually necessary. We now have some experience of managing patients who are completely ventilator-dependent with NIV, for example in the later stages of  Duchenne muscular dystrophy, and it is also possible to use NIV in some of these acute neurological diseases.  It is imperative that this is only done in a safe environment such as ICU.  The extent of muscle weakness should be re-evaluated regularly, paying particular attention to see if there is bulbar weakness.

**Key point**

Don't persevere with NIV too long in acute neurological syndromes – it is safer to intubate patients who are incapable of any spontaneous breathing or those with bulbar weakness.

## Summary

- NIV is a great treatment for type 2 respiratory failure in neuromuscular disorders
- Almost all of these patients will need NIV long term at home, often just at night
- NIPPV ventilation works better than BIPAP

# 24

# Volume Modes

## Learning points

By the end of this chapter you should be able to:

- Define tidal volume.
- Outline the difference between pressure- and volume-targeted NIV.
- *State the advantages of volume-targeted ventilation.*
- *State the disadvantages of volume-targeted ventilation.*

## Key words:

Volume-targeted ventilation

Up until now we have talked about target pressure: the same pressure is reached with each breath, but the amount of air entering the lungs with each breath (tidal volume) will vary - if the lungs are stiffer (less compliant), for the same pressure the tidal volume would become less:

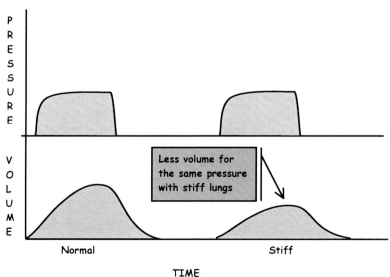

**Figure 24.1** Effect of compliance on tidal volume. If the target pressure remains the same but the lungs become stiffer – the breath on the right – the tidal volume will be less.

In volume-targeted ventilation a target tidal volume is set, and the ventilator uses as much pressure as is necessary to get that amount of air into the lungs; if the lungs get stiffer, it uses a higher pressure:

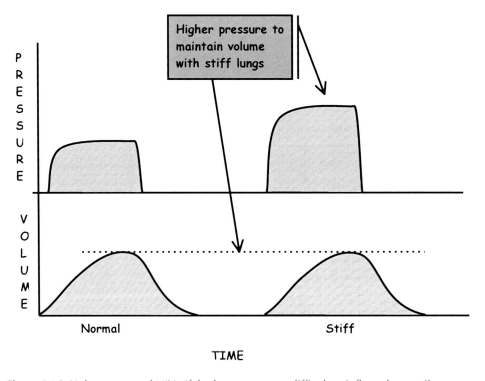

**Figure 24.2** Volume-targeted NIV. If the lungs are more difficult to inflate, the ventilator uses more pressure to ensure that the target tidal volume is achieved.

Caution is needed in using volume-controlled ventilation in the presence of a pneumothorax or in patients with bullous lung disease, where high pressures could be a problem. The advantage of this arrangement is that you are more certain of getting enough air into the lungs. This is certainly the case in a "closed" system such as an ICU ventilator attached to an endotracheal tube; if there is a leak in the system, as there invariably is around the mask in NIV, the advantage of setting volume is less obvious, because some of the volume is lost through the leaks. The evidence in favour of either volume- or pressure-targeted ventilation is not convincing, but there may be an advantage in switching from one to the other if your patient is not improving. Volume-targeted ventilation has been used for many years to ventilate neuromuscular patients at home. It works very well. Although there is an overwhelming trend towards the use of pressure-targeted modes, we should not forget that there will still be some patients who would be better on volume ventilators. Longer-established NIV centres tend to have more patients with neuromuscular conditions and are more likely to use volume-targeted ventilators.

## "Smart" volume modes

Ventilator manufacturers have started to combine the advantages of pressure- and volume-targeted modes. One example is AVAPS (average volume-assured pressure support). This is a servo mode of ventilation, whereby the ventilator alters what it does in response to changes in the patient's response. AVAPS tries to maintain tidal volume by increasing the inflation pressure. Another "smart" mode of ventilation is CS (for Cheyne-Stokes), which adapts to the cyclical changes in tidal volume and provides more pressure when the patient's effort reduces. The evidence so far is that these modes can provide more consistent ventilation. They seem to be well tolerated by patients. It remains to be seen whether in clinical practice there are substantial long-term benefits, or whether the greater sophistication compromises reliability.

## Summary

- Volume-controlled ventilation varies IPAP so that tidal volume is always the same.

- Smart modes of pressure-controlled ventilation attempt the same thing.

# 25
# Weaning

---

## Learning points

By the end of this chapter you should be able to:

- Describe when and how to extubate a patient and commence them on NIV.
- *Describe when and how to switch from tracheostomy ventilation to NIV.*
- *Wean a patient from NIV.*

## Keywords:

Weaning

---

Some patients don't breathe very well after an operation or general anaesthetic. Using NIV in these circumstances makes sense. There are still quite a few unanswered questions about which groups of patients it helps. We'll consider the different situations shortly, but what is clear is that if it is going to work you need to start it early.

> **Key points**
>
> If you are going to use NIV post-operatively, start it as soon as possible after extubation – don't wait until the patient runs into trouble, as it is much less likely to be effective at that stage.

## Weaning from endotracheal intubation to NIV

### Respiratory pump problems and elective surgical procedures

Patients with respiratory pump problems who have had elective surgical procedures – for example a gastroplasty, or insertion of a feeding enterostomy tube under general anaesthesia – are excellent candidates for post-operative NIV. Clearly if the patient is already using NIV long-term, they will need it immediately post-op.  There are some patients who are not yet at the stage of needing long-term NIV who will struggle post-operatively because of the effects of sedation, pain, analgesia, having to be supine etc.   This will usually be fairly easy to predict, and you can spend some time pre-operatively getting the patient used to NIV.  This will make things much easier post-op.  An example would be a patient with severe scoliosis, but without evidence of diurnal respiratory failure or nocturnal hypoventilation, who is going to undergo corrective spinal surgery.

Use NIPPV with an oro-nasal mask.  You may need a higher IPAP than you used in the pre-operative trial.  Depending on the type of operation, you may need to add supplementary oxygen.  Aim to use NIV continuously for the first 24 hours post-op, with increasing periods of spontaneous breathing during the next few days.  Clearly this will depend upon the type of operation and the speed of the patient's recovery.

### Early extubation

Most patients who have been ventilated invasively for any length of time, or in whom weaning delay is anticipated, will have had a tracheostomy.  This is fine most of the time, but weaning someone from ventilation via a tracheostomy to NIV takes time and sometimes you never manage it, for example in a patient with respiratory muscle weakness and a poor cough.  If you get the chance to go straight from intubation to NIV then it is well worth considering, provided the trial of NIV can be done safely.

I would opt for early extubation to NIV in patients with respiratory pump failure (muscle weakness, chest wall deformity, obesity-hypoventilation syndrome) who have been intubated and ventilated for an episode of severe acute respiratory failure, and whose blood gases rapidly return to normal.  The day after intubation you sometimes see patients who are easy to ventilate, with low inflation pressures, and who are easy to oxygenate on a fairly low inspired oxygen concentration.  This tells you that the lungs are in reasonable shape, and that the main problem on admission was the respiratory pump – muscle failure or a central drive problem.

The length of time patients with acute exacerbations of COPD need to be ventilated is sometimes surprisingly short.  You should think about transferring the patient onto NIV early, provided there is no evidence of pneumonia or other organ failure.   After extubation, some patients steadily deteriorate and need to be re-intubated.  In most instances the next step will be a tracheostomy.  You could have one more attempt at extubation, starting NIV straight away, provided this can be done safely.

Pre-requisites for transferring a patient to NIV are as follows:

- Normal $PaCO_2$.
- Normal arterial pH and bicarbonate.
- Normal, or only moderately low, $PaO_2$.
- Inspired oxygen concentration requirement less than 40%.
- Inflation pressure less than 30cm$H_2O$.

- Minimal respiratory tract secretions.

- Reasonable cough.

- Apyrexial.

- Stable cardiac rhythm.

- No inotropic support.

- Normal electrolytes.

- Stable renal function.

- No evidence of fluid overload.

- Functional gastro-intestinal tract.

- Adequate nutrition.

If all the above conditions are satisfied, there are a few questions to ask yourself:

- Will the patient wake up when you stop the sedation? We have already noted the dangers of NIV in impaired consciousness. An intubated patient you are thinking of extubating and starting on NIV is quite likely to be sedated. You will have to decide if they are likely to regain full consciousness after you stop the sedation. If not, then it will be safer to do a tracheostomy.

- Is it likely that the patient will be able to breath by themselves for at least a few minutes within the next 24 hours? Although the patient may need to be on NIV all the time initially, it is much safer if they are able to breathe spontaneously for at least a few minutes.

- Are the conditions optimal? You might decide to delay if it would be safer to extubate first thing the next morning, or at another time when the staffing arrangements are more secure, or when there is less going on elsewhere in ICU.

### *Practical Tip*

Extubate at a time of day when there is plenty of support at hand, and when the patient can be rapidly intubated again if NIV fails.

### *How to do it*

**Extubate and start NIV**

- Connect the NIV ventilator to the endotracheal tube for a few minutes to check that you are able to ventilate the patient effectively.
- Check that all the equipment needed for re-intubation is by the bedside.
- Select a suitable mask and straps.
- Turn sedation off, and wait for the patient to start waking up.

- Connect the NIV ventilator to the circuit and mask.
- Aspirate the nasogastic tube and remove it.
- Aspirate the pharynx.
- Aspirate the endotracheal tube.
- Remove the tube.
- Aspirate the pharynx again.
- Place the mask over the patient's face and start NIV.
- Wait a few minutes.
- Adjust the respiratory rate or IPAP on the ventilator if you need to.
- Strap the mask in place.

## Weaning to NIV from a tracheostomy

It is much more common to be weaning to NIV from a tracheostomy. First ask yourself if there is a reason why the tracheostomy should be left in place:

- Are you sure there is no anatomical problem with the upper airway?

- Does the patient have a good cough?

- Is the sputum volume so high that it is going to be easier to suction through a tracheostomy?

- Are there bulbar problems which may make swallowing unsafe?

- Is the patient going to be ventilator dependant 24 hours per day?

Then run through the list of pre-requisites we used for safe transfer from intubation to NIV.

***How to do it***

**Wean from a tracheostomy to NIV**

- Select a nasal mask and check that it fits comfortably on the patient.
- Connect the NIV ventilator you are going to use to the tracheostomy and check that is capable of ventilating the patient effectively.
- Disconnect the ventilator from the tracheostomy and connect it to the mask.
- Suction the trachea and pharynx.
- Deflate the cuff.
- Suction the trachea.
- Occlude the tracheostomy and check that the patient can breathe around the tracheostomy tube. If not, change the tube for a smaller one. You could use a fenestrated tube, but this is not essential.
- Attach the mask to the patient and commence NIV.
- If the chest does not expand, increase the IPAP.
- If the chest still does not expand, there is no connection between the upper airway

and the lungs. Re-connect the ventilator to the tracheostomy. Think about examining the cords with a fibreoptic scope. Change the tracheostomy for a smaller one.
- When the patient has been stable on NIV for 24 hours, remove the tracheostomy.
- Occlude the hole by placing a dressing over it. Cover this with two long pieces of elastic adhesive bandage in an X, extending up over the clavicles. Don't use "sleek" – it will soon blow off.
- If you are uneasy about removing the tracheostomy straight away, change it for a small cuffless tube.

## Weaning from NIV

The best way to wean from NIV is to gradually increase the length of periods of spontaneous breathing: this works better than turning down the pressure on the ventilator.

Stop NIV, and stay by the patient. Give them supplementary oxygen if they are likely to desaturate – this is quite safe just for a few minutes. Watch them breathe. Make sure they can achieve some chest expansion, particularly in patients with neuromuscular conditions – if not, restart NIV and think again. The respiratory rate may be high initially, but will fall within a few minutes. Don't put the patient back on the ventilator just because they look "tired" or anxious. Persevere, stay with them and they may settle down with reassurance.

The length of the first spontaneous breathing trial will vary. Some will only manage five minutes, but it is still an important step – make each subsequent trial slightly longer. Others will stay off for hours quite happily.

Put the patient back on full ventilation every night for the first few nights.

At this stage, always ask yourself if the patient might need nocturnal NIV, at least for a few months or possibly even in the long term. If you set up a respiratory support unit, you may well find that up to a third of patients presenting with acute respiratory failure end up going home on NIV.

*Key point*

To wean a patient from NIV, use progressively longer periods of spontaneous breathing, rather than reducing the pressures you use whilst they are on NIV.

There should be a daily plan, in which the amount of ventilatory support is reviewed and clear goals set. Every day you should ask yourself why your patient is still on a ventilator. Then decide what the minimum support they need is and make a plan accordingly. Aim low. You can always step back up if the patient starts to struggle - it is a common mistake to have patients on more support than they need.

*Practical Tip*

In patients with chronic lung disease, remember that their blood gases may be terrible even when they are stable and "well". If you aim for a normal $PaO_2$ it will take you ages to get them off ventilation.

The psychology of weaning is very important. It is easy for a patient with a tracheostomy on ICU to get downhearted. A few things that can make a difference are as follows:

- Make them feel more human again by enabling them to speak.

- See if it is possible for them to eat and drink.

- Improve the night-time environment so they get some sleep.

- Sit them out of bed.

- Get them dressed in their own clothes

- Remove as many tubes and probes as you can.

- A change of surroundings can work wonders; if you have the opportunity, move them from ICU to HDU or even a weaning centre.

In the journey towards ventilatory independence, there will be ups and downs. So long as the general trend is in the right direction, you need to help the patients cope with the bad days. Every day you should have specific targets, agreed on by you and the patient. If the previous day was disappointing for them, don't be too ambitious the next day. If you and the patient both believe that you will get there in the end, then your chances of getting there are high. If "you" is a different person every day, it will not be so easy.

*How to do it*

**Choose a tracheostomy tube to use with NIV**

When you are weaning a patient from invasive ventilation, you may need to change tracheostomy tubes more than once. Deciding which sort of tube to use can be confusing, so here are some tips:

- Use a cuffed tube to protect against aspiration if bulbar function is impaired or the patient has a poor cough reflex.
- Use a cuffed tube if the patient needs CPAP or BIPAP.
- Even with the cuff deflated, it can be difficult for the patient to breathe around a tracheostomy tube through their own upper airway.
- It is much easier to breathe around a smaller tracheostomy tube or an uncuffed tube.
- Use an uncuffed tube if the tracheostomy is only there to allow suction of secretions from the bronchial tree.
- A fenestration is a hole half way up the tracheostomy tube, through which the patient can breathe.
- Use a fenestrated tube when you want to block off the tracheostomy and get the patient to breathe through their upper airway – either spontaneously or with NIV.

- With a fenestrated tube, you will need to use an inner tube without a fenestration when you put a suction catheter down to aspirate secretions.
- Even with the cuff deflated and fenestration open, it can still be difficult to breathe through the upper airway.

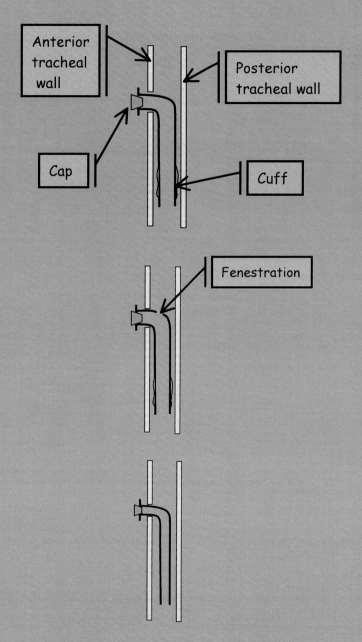

**Figure 25.1** Tracheostomy tubes. A: Cuffed - even with the cuff deflated, there may be very little room for the patient to breathe around the tube. B: Fenestrated - a hole allows communication with the upper airway; inner tubes come with and without fenestrations. C: Uncuffed - it is easier for the patient to breathe through their upper airway, particularly with a smaller diameter tube; fenestrated versions of uncuffed tubes are also available.

## Summary

- Don't miss an opportunity to try extubation directly to NIV in a patient with a respiratory pump problem.

- Extubation to NIV can be used in COPD, but be prepared to re-intubate as soon as it is apparent that you are going to struggle.

- If the patient needs nocturnal assisted ventilation only, consider changing from a tracheostomy to NIV.

# 26
# Physiotherapy

---

## Learning points

By the end of this chapter you should be able to

- Describe when NIV can help with expectoration.
- *Select patients with bronchiectasis who are suitable for NIV at home.*
- *Explain the difference between NIV and a cough-assist device.*

## Keywords:

Cough-assist.

---

For many years, physiotherapists have used positive-pressure devices to help with chest physiotherapy. NIV is no different in principle. NIV ventilators can be used to inflate the lungs fully to prevent basal collapse (atelectasis), or to increase the volume of air inspired before a cough in order to aid expectoration. The main indications are post-operative, bronchiectasis and neuromuscular problems.

## Intermittent NIV post operatively

Some patients may benefit from a short period of NIV every few hours or so in the immediate post-operative period. This is not an aid to weaning, but the sorts of patients will be similar:

- COPD.
- Obesity.
- Scoliosis.
- Neuromuscular disorders.

Patients with more severe disease who will be at increased risk of developing respiratory problems after surgery can be identified pre-operatively using spirometry and arterial blood gases.

Some operations are more likely to lead to respiratory complications:

- Thoracic surgery.
- Upper abdominal surgery.
- Spinal surgery.

Prevention is better than cure, so planning to use NIV post-op in high risk patients who undergo high-risk procedures is more likely to succeed than waiting until the patient is in trouble.

## Bronchiectasis

Evidence from studies in cystic fibrosis suggests that NIV is helpful in patients who desaturate during chest physiotherapy, in shortening the time it takes to recover from the physiotherapy session. It would seem reasonable to extrapolate this to bronchiectasis from other causes. It is unclear whether the volume of sputum expectorated is increased by the use of NIV.

NIV at night can help some patients with bronchiectasis. Their long term survival is poor, but NIV can reduce hospitalisation and improve their quality of life. In younger patients, it may just get them through to a lung transplant. Consider NIV in patients with bronchiectasis and the following:

- Young age.
- Severe disease.
- Frequent hospitalisations.
- Deteriorating blood gases despite optimal medical therapy.
- Hypercapnia.
- Good tolerance of NIV.

## Neuromuscular problems

NIV increases Vt. Inflation of the lower lobes of the lungs will be greater, which may prevent atelectasis. The prophylactic use of intermittent NIV in neuromuscular problems is debatable, but if the patient develops a chest infection then it can be very useful in conjunction with physiotherapy to aid expectoration of sputum.

**Cough**

There are three phases of cough:

*   Inspiration – inspiratory muscle contraction.
*   Compression – vocal cord closure, expiratory muscle contraction.
*   Expulsion – rapid vocal cord opening, expiratory muscle contraction.

An effective cough requires good function of the inspiratory, expiratory and vocal cord muscles. A good way of assessing this is to get the patient to cough into a peak flow meter. A peak cough flow of less than 270 litres/min implies that cough is ineffective and the patient may not be able to clear secretions from their lower respiratory tract if they develop an infection.

## Cough-assist devices

All the NIV we have discussed so far involves positive airway pressure. Cough assist devices apply positive pressure during inspiration, but then switch to a negative airway pressure during expiration. This produces higher expiratory flow rates than a positive pressure device alone, which helps with expectoration of secretions. These devices work well in patients with severe respiratory muscle weakness, particularly if they develop a chest infection and are struggling to expectorate secretions. Patients who are already using NIV often find that stepping up their daytime use of NIV is all that is required during a chest infection, without the additional expense of a cough-assist machine.

## NIV and rehabilitation

NIV can be used to help patients with COPD (and other respiratory diseases) do some exercise and build up their peripheral muscle strength. The patient, or a helper, can carry a battery-powered portable ventilator. Alternatively, a mains-powered ventilator can be used with a treadmill or exercise bicycle.

## Summary

*   NIV can be used as an adjunct to chest physiotherapy, post-operatively or in bronchiectasis.

*   A small proportion of patients with bronchiectasis benefit from NIV at home.

*   Cough-assist devices use negative pressure on the airway to increase expiratory flow rates.

# 27

# Chest wall problems

## Learning points

By the end of this chapter you should be able to:

- Describe how scoliosis affects breathing.
- Identify which patients with scoliosis need NIV.
- Manage patients with fractured ribs.
- *Recognize which patients with sequelae of tuberculosis (TB) might need NIV.*
- *Recognise which patients with polio might need NIV.*

## Keywords:

Scoliosis

## Scoliosis

There are two types of spinal curvature - kyphosis and scoliosis. In kyphosis, the spine is curved in only one plane, front to back. If you look from the side (or on a lateral CXR) the spine is curved forward, but if you look from the front or back the spine doesn't curve to one side or the other. Kyphosis has to be very severe to result in ventilatory failure, because the orientation of the ribs and the diaphragm remain fairly normal.

Scoliosis involves rotation of the spine, which looks curved if you view from either the side or the back. When the thoracic spine is scoliotic, the ribs are very distorted, and breathing is affected much more than in kyphosis. If the curvature is more than a right angle, then ventilatory failure is a risk. At this stage the VC will usually be less than 50% predicted. The curvature is also more likely to progress if the VC is under 50%.

Patients with scoliosis and a vital capacity under 50% predicted should have a clinical review and spirometry annually.

There are a few other risk factors for respiratory failure:

- If the patient has ever had spinal surgery then they are less likely to slip in to respiratory failure, possibly because the spine is more stable.

- If the scoliosis was present before the patient was five years old, then they will not have developed the normal complement of alveoli and are more likely to develop respiratory failure. Patients with congenital scoliosis should have an echocardiogram to check for associated cardiac defects.

- If the scoliosis is the result of weakness of the paraspinal muscles – from polio or muscular dystrophy – there will usually be associated respiratory muscle weakness and respiratory failure is much more common.

As with neuromuscular problems, hypercapnia first occurs at night, when ventilation is lower anyway. You identify nocturnal hypoventilation by overnight monitoring, but elevation of the daytime bicarbonate levels can also give you a clue. Many patients with severe scoliosis will underventilate for short periods during rapid eye movement (REM) sleep. You don't need to start NIV if the patient has no symptoms of sleep disturbance, but review the patient every 6 or 12 months and repeat the sleep study annually.

Once the daytime $PaCO_2$ is elevated, a crisis is just around the corner and the patient needs to be started on NIV; they may only need to have this at night, but they will need it for the rest of their lives. The prognosis for patients with scoliosis on NIV is excellent, with five year survival rates around 80%.

**Key point**

Patients with scoliosis who are hypercapnic need to be started on nocturnal NIV, irrespective of their pH.

## Mode of ventilation

NIPPV is the best mode, because you want to provide rather than support ventilation. (BIPAP is better than nothing if you can't get NIPPV organised immediately.) You will need to use an IPAP of at least 20cmH$_2$O, often more, to achieve adequate ventilation. The respiratory rate and I:E ratio should be set close to the patient's own spontaneous breathing pattern initially, to allow them to settle onto NIV and let the ventilator do the work of breathing for them.

Patients with scoliosis do worse in the longer term if they are hypoxic, have airflow obstruction or are very thin.

## Supplementary oxygen

After you start a patient on nocturnal NIV, their daytime blood gases will gradually improve over several months. The reasons for this slow improvement are not clear. As the daytime gases improve, so oxygenation overnight tends to pick up. Try and defer a decision about adding supplementary oxygen to NIV for at least six weeks after starting NIV. At that stage if the mean overnight oxygen saturation is less than 85%, add 2 litres/min and repeat the oximetry.

**Start a patient with chronic ventilatory failure on nocturnal NIPPV**

- Set up NIPPV.
- After a few minutes, stop NIV and make a plan with the patient.
- Aim for a short trial of NIV every hour in the daytime.
- Get the patient to go to bed on NIV that night.
- If after an hour they are unable to sleep, stop NIV, otherwise continue for as long as they can tolerate.
- If they weren't able to sleep on NIV, have further hourly trials the following day.
- Once they are able to sleep for at least four hours on NIV, monitor gas exchange overnight.

**Chest wall compliance**

The curve we looked at for compliance of the lungs showed an increase in their volume when positive pressure was applied to the airway. A similar curve could be drawn for the ribcage, when positive pressure is applied to the airway to inflate it above its resting (end-expiratory) level.

The lungs deflate fully when there is no pressure to inflate them. In contrast, the ribcage doesn't cave in completely when there is no pressure applied to the airway – you need to apply pressure to push it below its resting level. This pressure might be from the expiratory muscles, external pressure on the ribcage, or negative pressure on the airway. As with inflating the lungs or expanding the ribcage above its resting level, it becomes progressively more difficult to reduce the volume of the ribcage the further you get below the resting level:

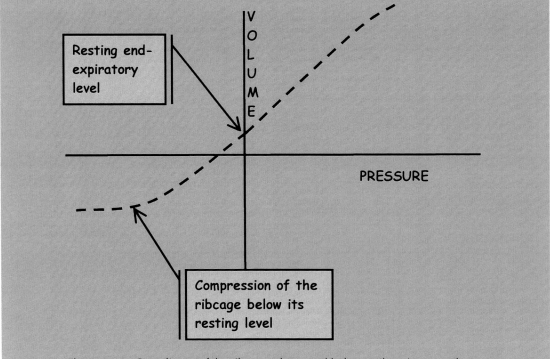

**Figure 27.1.** Compliance of the ribcage, above and below end-expiratory volume.

The compliance of the chest wall is such that in a normal subject it takes a pressure of about 10cmH$_2$O to get one litre of air in - this is similar to the compliance of the lungs. The pressure required to inflate the lungs <u>and</u> chest wall will be about 20cmH$_2$O for one litre of air - 10cmH$_2$O for the lungs and 10cmH$_2$O for the chest wall.

Note that the resting end-expiratory level for the chest wall is just above the intersection of pressure and volume. In vivo, the chest wall is pulled inwards to functional residual capacity (FRC) by the elastic recoil pressure of the lungs.

## Sequelae of tuberculosis

Prior to the discovery of anti-tuberculous chemotherapy, treatment for tuberculosis sometimes involved a phrenic nerve crush, artificial pneumothorax or thoracoplasty. These procedures, combined with the inevitable lung damage from the infection itself, left patients with a high work of breathing and/or impaired respiratory muscle pump. Many of these patients slip into hypercapnic respiratory failure as a late complication decades later. As with scoliosis, nocturnal NIV should be commenced if they are hypercapnic, irrespective of the pH level. NIV is reasonably effective at improving their clinical condition and blood gases, but long-term survival rates are poor. NIV should be set up as for scoliosis – the presence of airflow obstruction from endobronchial tuberculous scarring will usually require a slightly longer expiratory time. Supplementary oxygen is often necessary.

## Chest wall trauma

Multiple rib fractures are associated with a poor prognosis, particularly in the elderly. Aggressive pain management is essential if you are to avoid the patient developing pneumonia, and you may need invasive techniques such as intercostal blocks or an epidural.

> ### *Key points*
>
> Patients with fractured ribs do badly. Manage them on HDU and start BIPAP if they become hypercapnic.

BIPAP will keep the lungs inflated, and may reduce paradoxical motion of the ribcage, although good quality evidence for this is lacking. Get the patient onto HDU or ICU, watch carefully and start BIPAP at the first suggestion of trouble.

> ### *Physiology*
>
> **Flail segments**
>
> When a patient breathes in, there is a negative pressure within the chest – this is what causes the air to flow into the lungs. If the ribs are broken in two places, you may see that a segment of the ribcage moves inwards during inspiration. This is called a "flail" segment. Some of the energy used by the inspiratory muscles in generating a negative pressure is wasted by this flail motion. You can see inward motion of the ribcage during inspiration in some patients with scoliosis or after a thoracoplasty.

## Polio

Before the introduction of vaccination, polio was a common cause of ventilatory failure. Much of what we know today about ventilation was learnt during polio epidemics. Some patients have been ventilated continuously at home since the 1950s. From time to time you will probably come across patients with polio who slip into ventilatory failure many years after their original illness. The reasons for this late deterioration are not clear; it could be that the non-affected muscles are subject to normal ageing processes, having had years of coping with an increased load. Patients with polio you need to keep a close eye on are:

- Patients who needed artificial ventilation (such as an iron lung) during the acute illness.
- Those with a thoracic scoliosis, following paraspinal muscle paralysis.
- Upper limb polio.
- Vital capacity less than 50% predicted.

NIV works well in polio. Use nocturnal NIPPV. You may need quite high inspiratory pressures 20–30cmH$_2$O or even higher. As with scoliosis, think about adding supplementary oxygen if after a couple of months of nocturnal NIV the mean SpO$_2$ overnight is less than 85%.

---

### Practical Tip

If you order oxygen for patients with chronic hypercapnic respiratory failure on NIV, tell the patient to use it only when they are on NIV at night and not during the day. It is not like long-term oxygen therapy in COPD, which should be used for 12 or 15 hours per day – supplementary oxygen without NIV can be dangerous in patients with chest wall problems, as in other causes of chronic type 2 respiratory failure, because it removes hypoxic drive.

---

### Physiology

**Improvement in daytime blood gases with nocturnal NIV**

When you start a patient on NIV, their daytime arterial blood gases – both PaO$_2$ and PaCO$_2$ – tend to get steadily better over several months. Why? Well, the possibilities include:

- The breathing muscles get stronger, because they get a rest at night.
- The lungs and/or ribcage get easier to move (more compliant), because of the action of the ventilator at night.
- Respiratory drive picks up.

The answer appears to be respiratory drive. Maximum mouth pressures, vital capacity, etc, don't change much but respiratory drive picks up. The reasons for this are not clear, but correction of nocturnal hypoventilation is likely to be the most important factor, "resetting" respiratory drive back to more normal blood gas values than those to which they had become accustomed.

---

## Summary

- Patients with scoliosis of sufficient severity to reduce VC below 50% predicted are at risk of type 2 respiratory failure.
- If the daytime PaCO$_2$ is elevated, start long-term nocturnal NIV.
- Use pressure-controlled ventilation: NIPPV.
- Use these principles to manage patients with sequelae of TB or polio.
- Use BIPAP for patients with multiple rib fractures.

# 28

# Long-Term

---

## Learning points

By the end of this chapter you should be able to:

- Make a list of the types of patient who might need NIV at home.
- *Teach a patient the skills they need to set up their ventilator.*
- *Discharge a patient home safely on NIV.*
- *Outline how you would follow them up.*

---

Most of this book has been about acute NIV. We have strayed into some areas which are more relevant to the long-term. You may become interested in home NIV if you have a patient who presented in acute respiratory failure but is now better and needs to continue with NIV in the long term. You may have come across out-patients who are slipping into chronic respiratory failure and need to start NIV electively. You are likely to send these patients to a regional unit, but might like to know a little more, particularly if you are going to provide the local bit of a "shared care" package.

> ### Key points
>
> About half of the patients who use NIV long-term at home start this after an emergency admission to hospital with acute respiratory failure.

I am not going to cover all aspects of long-term NIV: there are several excellent books on the topic, details of which are in the bibliography. There is no one right way of setting up home NIV, and very little high quality evidence on which to base recommendations.

## Patients

Most home ventilation services have a large proportion of patients with either neuromuscular problems or obesity-hypoventilation syndrome.   There are probably still quite a few patients with these diseases who would benefit from long-term NIV but are not offered it.  Smaller numbers of patients will have scoliosis.  A few will have long-term sequelae of poliomyelitis or tuberculosis.  The number of patients with airway diseases on NIV at home is very variable, and alarmingly high in some countries given the absence of evidence of benefit for long term-NIV in these patients at the present time.

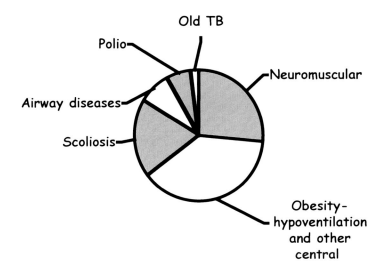

**Figure 28.1** Aetiology of respiratory failure for adult patients on long-term ventilation in Nottingham.

It may seem obvious that the reason why the patient went into respiratory failure should be established, but it is easy to forget to do this if the patient came in with acute respiratory failure and was too unwell to do many tests on admission.

### *Practical Tip*

Check that spirometry, mouth pressures etc have all been documented, and that other tests such as imaging have been completed before discharge. Get an up-to-date daytime arterial blood gas. Make sure that NIV provides adequate ventilation overnight.

## NIV Competency

Get the patient to decide what they need to know about NIV.  You can offer some choices and guidance, but it is much better if they make decisions about what they want to learn rather than you.  Make a list.  Prioritise – start with the really important issues.  You will be able to build on their knowledge and skills over time.  The initial list for a patient with obesity-hypoventilation syndrome, for example, might be:

- What is wrong with my breathing?
- Why do I need a ventilator?
- How do I fit the mask?
- How do I turn the ventilator on?
- How do I keep the equipment clean?
- Who do I contact if I have a problem?

There are some key principles about any form of teaching:

- Active is better than passive learning – it is imperative that you get the person you are teaching to do things.
- Assume nothing – it is easy to forget to explain something that is second nature to you, for example something simple like turning the ventilator on.
- Less is more – don't teach too much in one session.  Break things down into small manageable chunks.
- Context/content/closure – explain why you need to teach the topic (for example, washing the mask), teach it, then summarise what has been learnt.  Ideally the learner should do the summarising, which allows you to check that you have got the message across.  This can be a bit depressing when they can't explain what you have so painstakingly taught them, but it is better you know that you have failed.

***How to do it***

**Teach a patient or carer a practical skill**

- Explain what you are going to teach.
- Explain why they need to know.
- Demonstrate the skill, talking through each step along the way.
- Demonstrate the skill again, but remain silent whilst you do so.
- Perform the skill again, but this time in response to instructions from the patient/carer.  If they give you the wrong instruction, don't carry it out; explain what the consequences would be if you did, then give the correct step.  If you need to correct any instructions, you ought to repeat the whole skill again.
- Get the patient/carer to demonstrate the skill to you.  If they need prompts, repeat the whole skill one more time.
- Document what you have taught.

## Equipment

Clearly the patient needs to know how to switch their ventilator on and off, and again be able to demonstrate this to you. It is unlikely that you will need the patient or their carers to adjust the ventilator settings at this stage, although some do when they are more conversant with NIV. Even if the ventilator allows you to lock the controls, it is good practice to write the settings down – keep one copy and put another in the folder the patient is going to take home with them.

Circuits have a habit of becoming disconnected from ventilators when they are moved around, so a diagram of what goes where is essential. In addition to being able to put on their mask properly, the patient needs to be able to take the mask apart for washing, and to re-assemble it. Cleanliness rather than sterility is the message for infection control at home. Equipment that looks clean is fine. Visibly dirty masks and circuits will be colonised by a variety of micro-organisms, although surprisingly these seldom cause clinical infections. A daily wash in warm soapy water is best for masks, with a weekly wash in a dishwasher. Careful drying is important. Circuits should be cleaned about once every two weeks, ideally by putting them in an ordinary dishwasher. Alternatively, hot water and detergent can be used. The circuit should be dissembled into its component parts before washing, particularly the exhalation valve. It is important to hang the circuits up to dry thoroughly after washing. A weekly wipe down with a damp cloth or wipe will usually be sufficient to keep the ventilator clean.

You may also need to think about spare ventilators, back-up power supplies or a self-inflating resuscitation bag for emergencies in patients who are very dependent on NIV.

## Written instructions

All this needs to be written down, for the patient or their carers to refer to when they are at home. You may choose to give them the instruction booklet for their ventilator, the leaflets that come with the masks and so on, but you need to summarise the important information. You could make up a folder for the patient with

- A diagram of how to put the mask on.
- Details of the type and size of mask, in case it needs replacing.
- A diagram of how the circuit fits together.
- How to turn the ventilator on.
- Table of ventilator settings.
- Action to take if the alarms go off.
- Emergency contact number.

## Follow-up

> **Key point**
>
> Tailor follow-up to the individual patient.

The longer the patient has been in hospital, the more stressful returning home is likely to be. In some cases it may be best to arrange a visit at home later that day. At the very minimum, a telephone call the next day will be needed, followed-up by a home visit if necessary. We usually see the patient or at home within one week. They have another out-patient appointment in another month, and three-monthly thereafter. After a year, in very stable patients we sometimes push this interval up to 6 months. After another couple of years we may opt for annual appointments, provided the patient is happy with this and knows what to do if they have a problem.

## Summary

- Long-term NIV at home is an excellent treatment for patients with type 2 respiratory failure as a result of scoliosis, neuromuscular diseases or obesity.

# Bibliography

Disorders of ventilation. John Shneerson. Blackwell Scientific Publications, Oxford 1988. ISBN 0-632-01668-X.

Noninvasive Mechanical Ventilation. John R. Bach. Hanley and Belfus, Philadelphia 2002. ISBN 1-56053-549-0.

Non-invasive Positive Pressure Ventilation: Principles and Applications. Nicholas S. Hill (ed). Futura, New York 2001. ISBN 0-87993-459-X.

Non-invasive Respiratory Support. A Practical Handbook. Anita K. Simmonds (ed). Arnold, London 2001. ISBN 0-340-76259.

# Index

*For kt*